ATLAS ON THE
SURGICAL ANATOMY
OF LARYNGEAL CANCER

ATLAS ON THE SURGICAL ANATOMY OF LARYNGEAL CANCER

JOHN A. KIRCHNER, MD

Professor Emeritus, Otolaryngology
Department of Surgery
Yale University School of Medicine

SINGULAR PUBLISHING GROUP, INC.
SAN DIEGO · LONDON

Singular Publishing Group, Inc.
401 West A Street, Suite 325
San Diego, California 92101-7904

Singular Publishing Group, Ltd.
19 Compton Terrace
London N1 2UN, UK

Singular Publishing Group, Inc., publishes textbooks, clinical manuals, clinical reference books, journals, videos, and multimedia materials on speech-language pathology, audiology, otorhinolaryngology, special education, early childhood, aging, occupational therapy, physical therapy, rehabilitation, counseling, mental health, and voice. For your convenience, our entire catalog can be accessed on our website at **http//www.singpub.com.** Our mission to provide you with materials to meet the daily challenges of the everchanging health care/educational environment will remain on course if we are in touch with you. In that spirit, we welcome your feedback on our products. Please telephone **(1-800-521-8545),** fax **(1-800-774-8398),** or e-mail **(singpub@mail.cerfnet.com)** your comments and requests to us.

Typeset in 10/12 Palatino by Thompson Type
Printed in Hong Kong by Paramount Printing

Library of Congress Cataloging-in-Publication Data
Kirchner, John A., 1915–
    Atlas on the surgical anatomy of laryngeal cancer / John A. Kirchner.
     p. cm.
    ISBN 1-56593-776-7
    1. Larynx—Cancer—Surgery—Atlases.   2. Larynx—Anatomy—Atlases.
3. Larynx—Histopathology—Atlases.   4. Anatomy, Surgical and
topographical—Atlases. I. Title.
    [DNLM: 1. Laryngeal Neoplasms—surgery—atlases. 2. Larynx—
anatomy & histology—atlases.   WV 17 K58a 1998]
RF516.K56   1998
616.99'422059—dc21
DNLM/DLC
for Library of Congress
                              97-45063
                                 CIP

CONTENTS

FOREWORD

During the 25 year period 1964 through 1989, Dr. John Kirchner studied 442 total and partial laryngectomy specimens by whole-organ serial sections. His findings are not merely descriptive, but are presented from the viewpoint of a surgeon looking for answers to clinical problems in his patients. As a result, the study has produced a wealth of information about the growth and spread of laryngeal cancer. In numerous publications derived from this work, he has reported insights on the prognosis, behavior, and treatment of various laryngeal and hypopharyngeal cancers that have created a basis for current surgical management of these tumors.

In *Atlas on the Surgical Anatomy of Laryngeal Cancer,* Dr. Kirchner has selected 70 of the 442 specimens and assembled them into a concise yet comprehensive synopsis of the spectrum of laryngeal cancers commonly encountered in clinical practice. The information is invaluable for surgeons, oncologists, radiologists, and pathologists at all levels of experience. The impact of the vivid photomicrographs is breathtaking, providing a level of understanding of the intra- and extralaryngeal spread of tumor not possible by any other method of analysis. The surgical specimens, their corresponding sections, and the clinical resumés illustrate the suitability or unsuitability of various types of surgical or irradiation therapy.

Features of laryngeal cancer demonstrated in the sections include the containment of early cancers by fibroelastic barriers within the larynx; clinically inapparent framework invasion and extralaryngeal spread associated with tumors that deeply infiltrate the paraglottic space; mechanisms of vocal cord fixation in glottic cancer; the occasional transglottic spread of supraglottic cancer; and the persistence of tumor beneath apparently intact mucosa in irradiation failures. The safe margins attained with partial laryngectomy for many large supraglottic tumors are illustrated. Fixed-cord glottic tumors amenable to partial laryngectomy are shown, and the need for more extensive resection in other types is demonstrated

It is unlikely that a similar collection of whole-organ sections will be amassed in the future. Except for endoscopic laser resection, total and partial laryngectomy for early laryngeal cancers are being used less frequently. For advanced tumors, the various chemotherapy and irradiation protocols being employed in many centers will result in fewer previously untreated specimens.

This volume will provide a continuing source of detailed information on the behavior of laryngeal cancer. It is a contemporary classic that will grace the bookshelves of clinicians and institutions for generations to come.

Carl E. Silver, MD
Professor of Surgery
Professor of Otolaryngology
Albert Einstein College of Medicine
Chief, Head and Neck Surgery
Bronx, New York

PREFACE

Despite significant advances during recent years in irradiation and medical oncology, primary surgical treatment continues to offer the best hope of local control for certain types of laryngeal cancer. For glottic tumors with limited mobility, for example, conservation surgery has resulted in local controls that exceed those obtained by radiotherapy. Supraglottic cancer with invasion of the preepiglottic space is controlled in most cases by supraglottic resection, whereas cancer in this poorly vascularized, fat-filled space presents a difficult problem for the radiotherapist.

The present study was undertaken in 1965 in an effort to determine whether total laryngectomy was unnecessarily radical for fixed-cord glottic lesions and for supraglottic cancer invading the preepiglottic space. By 1989 a total of 442 surgical specimens had been processed from our practice at Yale-New Haven Hospital. Of this group, 70 have been selected for this volume as representing behavior typical of squamous cell cancer in various parts of the larynx and hypopharynx. The surgical specimens and corresponding sections provide the rationale for various forms of conservation surgery of the larynx.

I am grateful to the 48 of my patients whose surgical specimens appear in this study. Members of our staff supplied the remaining 22 specimens from their own patients, 10 from Dr. Clarence T. Sasaki, 3 from Dr. W. J. Goodwin, 2 each from Drs. H. R. Pillsbury, J. R. Loeffler, E. Yanagisawa, and R. Rosnagle, and 1 from Dr. Gordon Strothers.

I am deeply indebted to our chairman, Dr. Clarence T. Sasaki, for persuading me to organize and display the results of my quarter-century study of partial and total laryngectomy specimens. After my retirement from clinical practice in 1985 he provided me with an office furnished with modern communication equipment including computerized access to descriptions of the 442 serially sectioned specimens that make up the present collection. The sections are stored in a room adjoining my office, where they can be studied and photographed. Without Dr. Sasaki's support and encouragement I would not have undertaken this project, nor would I have been able to carry it to completion.

In assembling working prints of selected specimens, I was fortunate in obtaining advice from the master of photodocumentation, Doctor Eiji Yanagisawa. It was he who convinced me that although many details of individual specimens and sections were obvious to me, they might be less so to others seeing the material for the first time. I have, therefore, added arrows and labels to some of the photographs while trying to avoid covering the essentials.

Long before the manuscript was sent to the editor, each section was scrutinized word for word by my son, J. Cameron Kirchner, MD. It was his insistence on clarity that persuaded me to write several drafts of the manuscript before sending it to the publisher for final editing. Despite a heavy clinical practice, Cameron spent the necessary time and effort to ferret out ambiguities and jargon and to identify points that might not have been clear to the reader.

I was very fortunate, early in the project, to obtain the services of an expert in celloidin sections, Mrs. Sylvia Freeman. She used hematoxylin and eosin the way an artist uses oil paint or watercolors. Her standards were high and always consistent. Any section that was not completely wrinkle-free when mounted on the slide was disqualified for further use and condemned to the trash bin.

Since its inception, this study was supported by generous grants from the National Cancer Institute, United States Public Health Service.

Many of the specimens have been previously displayed, in small numbers, in textbooks and journals. To the best of my knowledge these have all been acknowledged in the text.

How my dear wife, Aline, survived the disarray I created in our home with piles of reprints, journals, slides, and books on tables, chairs, and windowsills is beyond my comprehension. For this and many other evidences of her support I shall be eternally grateful.

To Aline
Merci pour tout

INTRODUCTION

The surgeon who performs any type of partial laryngectomy must be able to predict the margins of safety and the possibility of preserving the protective mechanism of the residual larynx. The radiotherapist, on the other hand, must estimate tumor volume and the likelihood of anoxic cells within the lesion. Modern imaging techniques facilitate these assessments, but are limited by variations in framework ossification, by movement artifacts, and by infection deep within the soft tissues. Nor can modern imaging reveal, in precise detail, the fibroelastic membranes and ligaments that form the boundaries of the intralaryngeal compartments within which cancer is confined in its early stages and that make conservation surgery possible. Surgical specimens and whole-organ sections of laryngectomy specimens provide the basis for interpreting clinical findings and the images obtained by preoperative MRI and radiographic techniques.

Total or partial laryngectomy was the primary treatment for most specimens in this atlas. Five radiotherapy failures are included to show the usual sites of residual or recurrent cancer. Three other laryngectomy specimens, treated with 4000r in a combined protocol, show the difficulty in assessing tumor margins at operation. In none of the patients had chemotherapy been administered before surgery.

In most cases the surgical specimen was sectioned in a plane determined by the tumor's location. Glottic and transglottic tumors were sec-tioned in the coronal plane to show the tumor's relation to the ventricle, the extent of its infraglottic spread, and the presence or absence of framework invasion. Most supraglottic tumors were sectioned sagitally to show the relationship to the anterior commissure, preepiglottic space, hyoid bone, and base of the tongue. Pyriform sinus lesions were usually sectioned transversely to show the relationship to the posterior aspect of the cricoid plate, posterior cricoarytenoid muscle, paraglottic space, and supraglottic larynx.

After the laryngectomy specimen is opened, the surgeon's first view of the tumor is from its posterior aspect. For this reason, whole-organ sections in this volume are oriented in the same way, with right-sided tumor appearing on the right side of the photograph in coronal sections. Transverse sections are shown as viewed from above, whereas in sagittal sections the endolarynx faces left or right, depending on the side of tumor involvement. A schema in the lower corner of each photograph explains the orientation and plane of the section.

Although the terms "dorsal" and "ventral" are appropriate when used in Comparative Anatomy, the human's upright position has resulted in these terms being replaced by "posterior" and "anterior." For the same reason, "cephalad" and "caudal" are expressed as "upper" and "lower" or "superior" and "inferior" in modern reports. The latter terminology is followed in this volume. "Transverse" is the plane at right angles to the long axis of the larynx.

Review-type articles were selected when available, and reports illustrating original operations are cited whenever possible. Several recent reports, not identified as reviews, bring the status of an operation up to date and provide references to the original report.

GLOTTIC CANCER

In assessing glottic cancer for its suitability for partial laryngectomy the surgeon must determine the tumor's size; its extent below the glottic level; mobility of the true vocal cord; the tumor's surface appearance, whether exophytic or ulcerated; and its relationship to the arytenoid cartilage, ventricle, anterior commissure, and base of the epiglottis. Submucosal induration often reveals invasion beyond the tumor's visible limits.

These physical characteristics reflect the extent of a tumor's deeper component and the likelihood that it has invaded the laryngeal framework (thyroid and cricoid cartilages). Invasion of the framework is one of the factors related to local control of the disease and to disease-free survival time.[1]

It is not clear whether the perichondrium alone or perichondrium in combination with the underlying cartilage is the real barrier. Nevertheless, the perichondrium, which by definition overlies cartilage, appears to be a more effective barrier when it overlies the unossified parts of the same framework. These and other relationships are demonstrated in the following surgical specimens and their whole-organ sections.

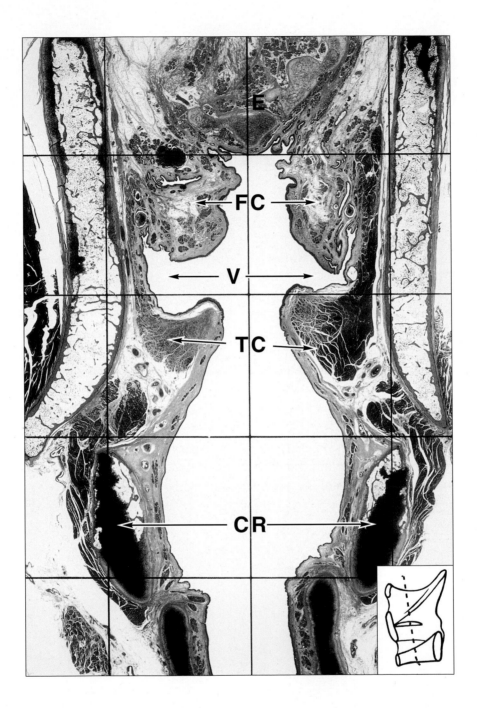

PLATE 1. Coronal section, mid-larynx, adult male. The 1-cm grid shows that the upper edge of the cricoid cartilage (CR) is about 1 cm below the free edge of the true vocal cord (TC). This dimension is valid only in the mid-larynx area. The lower edge of the thyroid and upper edge of the cricoid cross at this plane, located at the same coronal plane as the inferior thyroid tubercle. The thickness of the thyroid cartilage increases from anterior to posterior, with its maximum at the oblique line.[2] The paraglottic space is not prominent in this section, but is present as a thin strip along the inner surface of the thyroid ala above and below the ventricular fundus (cf. Plate 67). V = ventricle FC = false cord

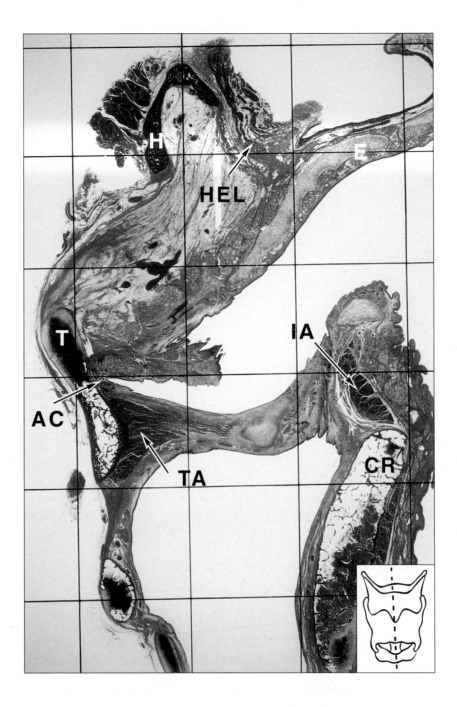

PLATE 2. Midsagittal section, adult male larynx with 1-cm grid. The lower edge of the thyroid cartilage (T) lies about 1 cm below the anterior commissure (AC) and has undergone ossification. The anterior portion of the cricoid cartilage is seen at about 17 mm below the commissure, whereas in the posterior larynx the top of the cricoid plate (CR) lies only a few millimeters below the glottic level. The top of the cricoid cartilage serves as the lower line of resection in conventional vertical hemilaryngectomy[3] and in the various forms of supracricoid laryngectomy.[4] The dimension is important in resecting anterior commissure lesions with downward extension and should not be exceeded. H = hyoid bone HEL = hyoepiglottic ligament E = epiglottis IA = interarytenoid muscle TA = thyroarytenoid muscle (Reprinted from Kirchner, JA. Vertical Partial Resections of the Larynx—Posttherapeutic Histology, Microstaging. In: Wigand ME, Steiner W, Stell PM, eds. *Functional Partial Laryngectomy* [Fig 2, p 128]. New York: Springer-Verlag, © 1984, with permission.)

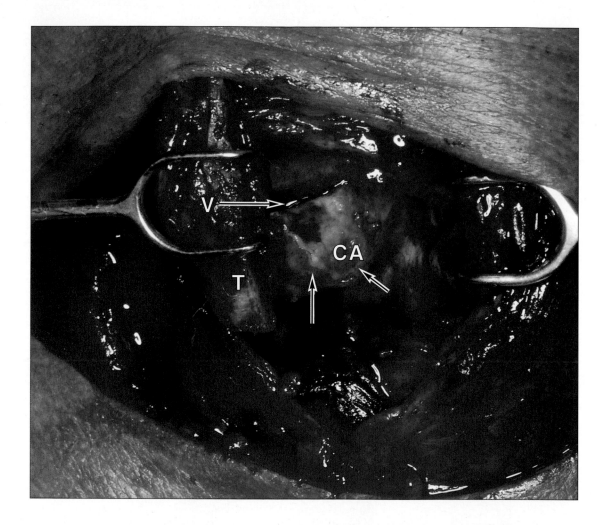

PLATE 3. Thyrotomy exposure for vertical hemilaryngectomy. A saw cut has been made in the thyroid cartilage (T) to the left of the midline. The tumor (CA) of the right true cord does not cross the ventricle (V), nor does it extend more than 1 cm below the glottic level. Lower arrows indicate lower edge of the tumor.

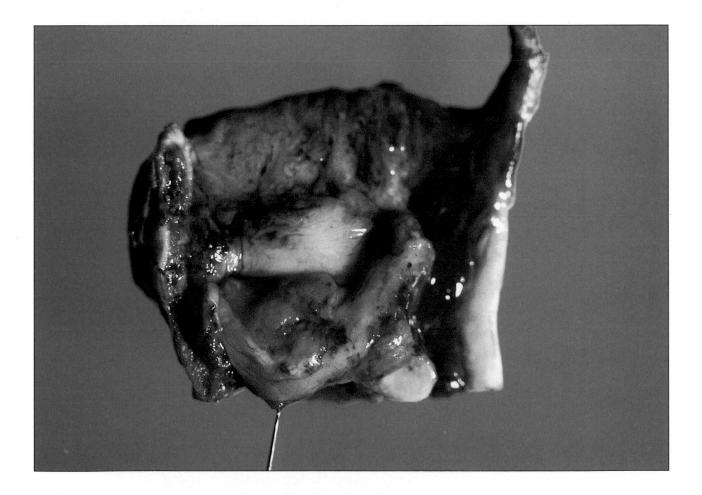

PLATE 4. The vertical hemilaryngectomy specimen shows an adequate lower margin, the resection having been made along the edge of the cricoid cartilage. The vocal cord was mobile on preoperative laryngoscopy, but the anterior commissure was difficult to evaluate.

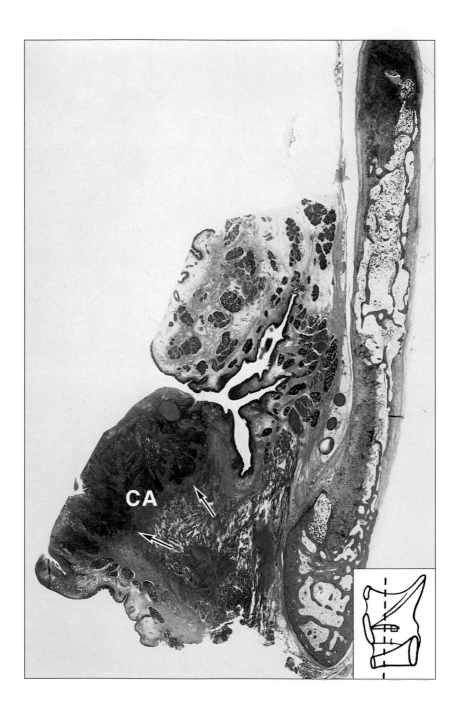

PLATE 5. Coronal section of the previous specimen. Free mobility of the true cord indicates little or no invasion of the underlying musculature and probable suitability for radiotherapy. Arrows indicate the tumor (CA) margin. (Reprinted from Kirchner JA. Vertical Partial Resections of the Larynx—Posttherapeutic Histology, Microstaging. In: Wigand ME, Steiner W, Stell PM, eds. *Functional Partial Laryngectomy* [Fig 3, p 129]. New York: Springer-Verlag, © 1984, with permission.)

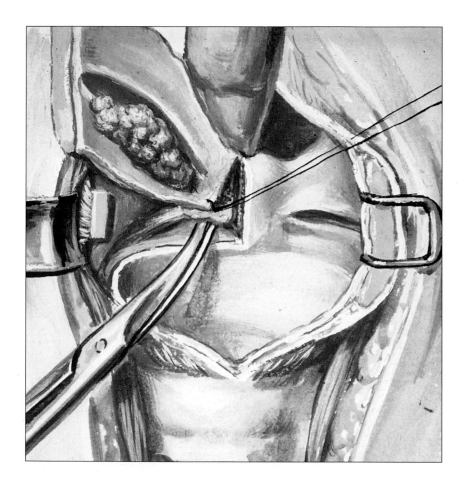

PLATE 6. Frank Netter's drawing of hemilaryngectomy.[3] The surgical specimen has been mobilized inferiorly by sharp dissection along the top of the cricoid cartilage. Scissors are now being used to cut across the base of the vocal process. If the body of the arytenoid requires removal, the area should be reconstructed to prevent aspiration.[5]

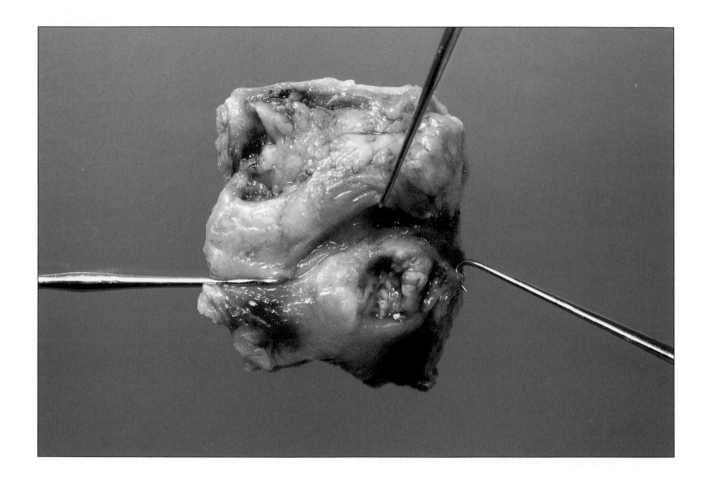

PLATE 7. Hemilaryngectomy specimen, glottic carcinoma with limited mobility. The hook on the right side indicates anterior commissure. Tumor has destroyed the free edge of the true cord. Margins are grossly adequate. Limited mobility in a glottic tumor may be due to bulk alone or to invasion of the underlying musculature.

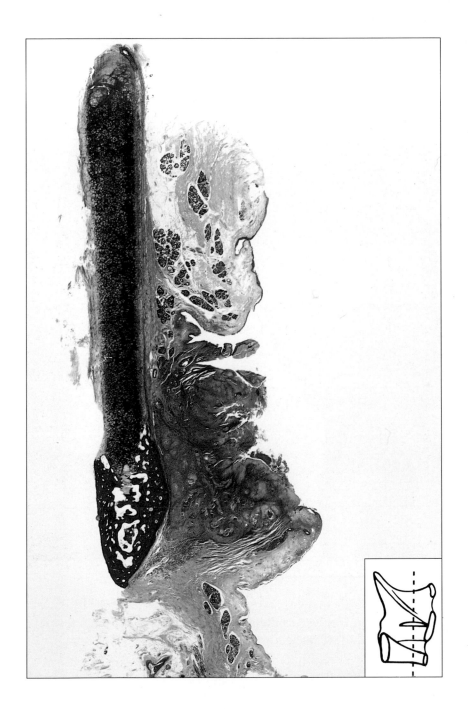

PLATE 8. Moderate invasion of the thyroarytenoid muscle in the previous surgical specimen. Good inferior margin. Glottic lesions with limited mobility have not responded well to radiotherapy.

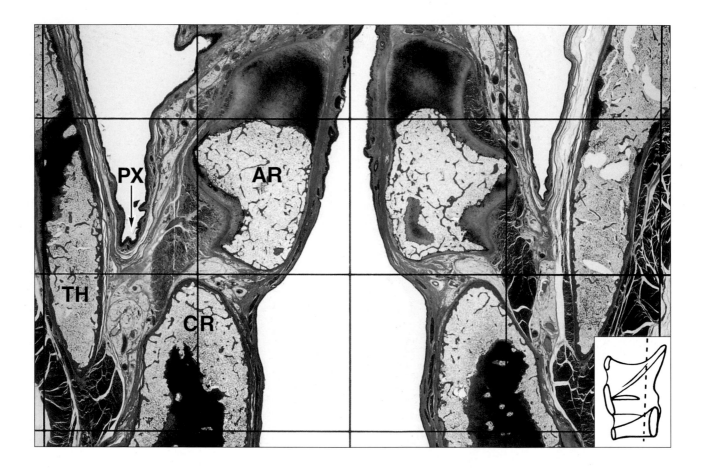

PLATE 9. Coronal section, normal larynx, at arytenoid area (AR), 1-cm grid. The top of the cricoid ring (CR) in the posterior larynx lies within millimeters of the glottic level as indicated by the arytenoid cartilage. PX = pyriform sinus apex TH = thyroid cartilage

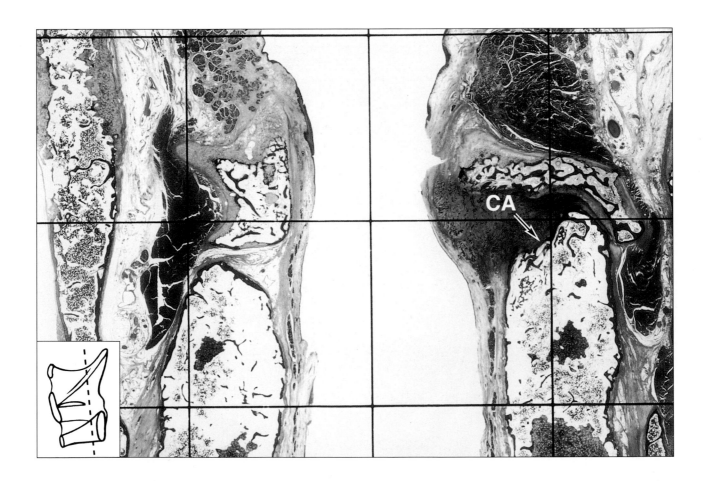

PLATE 10. Coronal section of glottic cancer, posterior part of larynx. 1-cm grid. Cancer (CA) extends 3 or 4 mm below glottic level and has begun to invade the top of the cricoid plate. (Reprinted from Kirchner JA. The Systems of UICC and AJC for Staging of Laryngeal Carcinoma. In: Wigand ME, Steiner W, Stell PM, eds. *Functional Partial Laryngectomy* [Fig 3, p 72]. New York: Springer-Verlag, © 1984, with permission.)

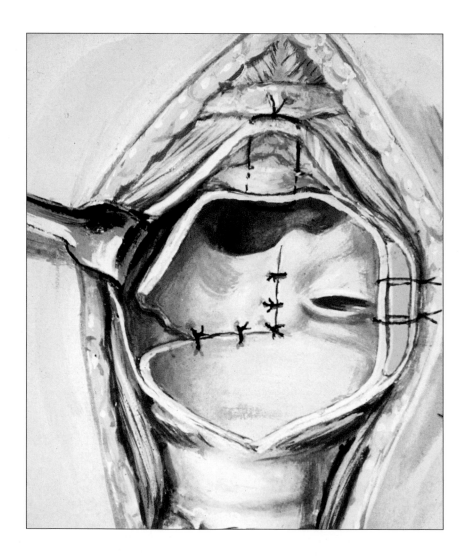

PLATE 11. Frank Netter's drawing of closure after hemilaryngectomy.[3] The arytenoid in this case has been removed and the defect merely resurfaced with mucosa advanced from the pyriform sinus. This technique leaves the pyriform sinus with a shallow or nonexistent fundus that allows direct access of liquids into the trachea.

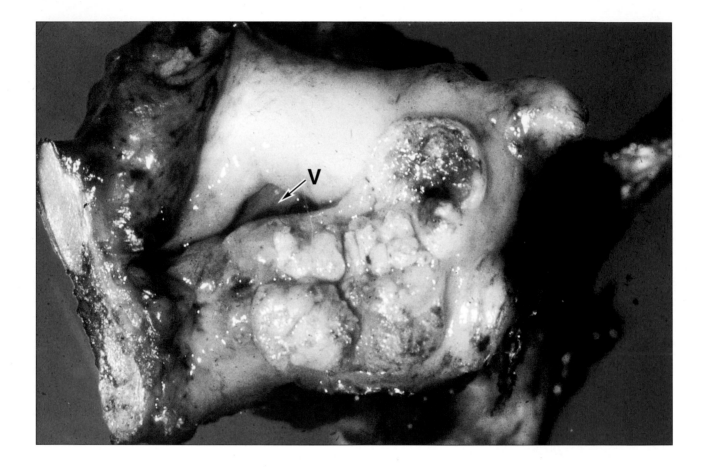

PLATE 12. Hemilaryngectomy specimen, right glottic cancer. Preoperative laryngoscopy showed limited mobility of the true cord. Carcinoma extending upward behind the ventricle required resection of the arytenoid cartilage. The defect was not reconstructed, but resurfaced with mucosa advanced from the pyriform sinus. Postoperatively, the patient reported frequent aspiration of cold liquids. Hot liquids, however, which he sipped slowly, rarely produced aspiration. V = ventricle (Reprinted from Kirchner, JA, Carter D. The Larynx. In: Sternberg SS, ed. *Diagnostic Surgical Pathology* 2nd ed [Fig 15]. New York: Raven Press, © 1994, with permission.)

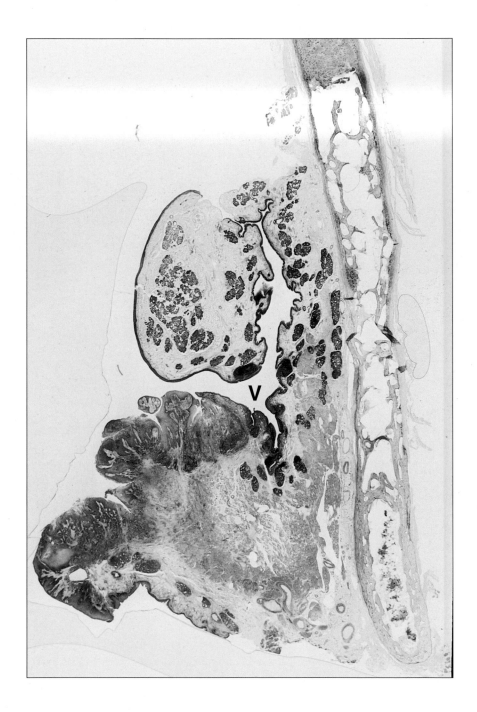

PLATE 13. Coronal section of the previous specimen. Carcinoma extends laterally along the floor of the ventricle (V) without invading the glottic musculature. Limited mobility of the cord may sometimes be due entirely to this type of extension. As seen in the gross specimen, however, tumor at the arytenoid cartilage may be an additional reason for limited mobility. (Reprinted from Kirchner JA. Vertical Partial Resections of the Larynx—Posttherapeutic Histology, Microstaging. In: Wigand ME, Steiner W, Stell PM, eds. *Functional Partial Laryngectomy* [Fig 5, p 129]. New York: Springer-Verlag, © 1984, with permission.)

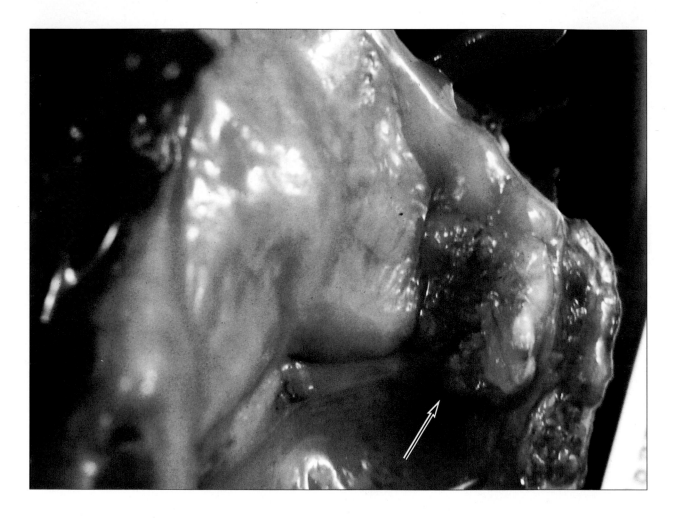

PLATE 14. Total laryngectomy specimen. The patient was a 78-year-old woman complaining of hoarseness and right-sided sore throat. Most of the visible tumor occupied the arytenoid area above, below, and behind the ventricle. The true cord showed moderately impaired mobility, with tumor extending to its posterior end (arrow).

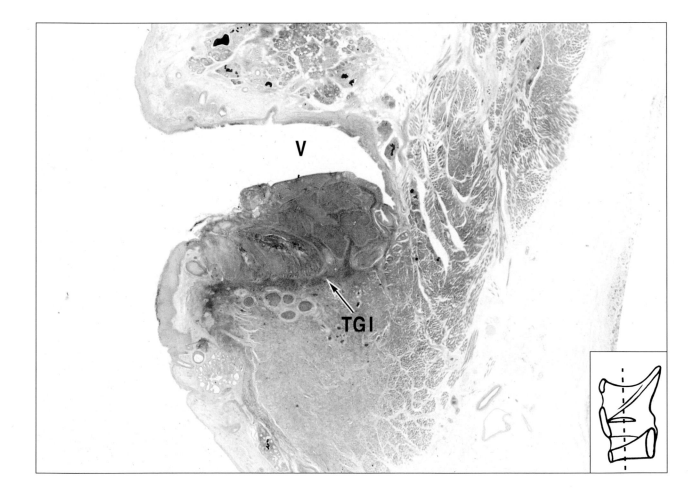

PLATE 15. Coronal section of the previous specimen through right mid-larynx. Tumor occupies the surface of the true cord along the floor of the ventricle (V). Small nests of cancer are present below the thyroglottic ligament (TGl).

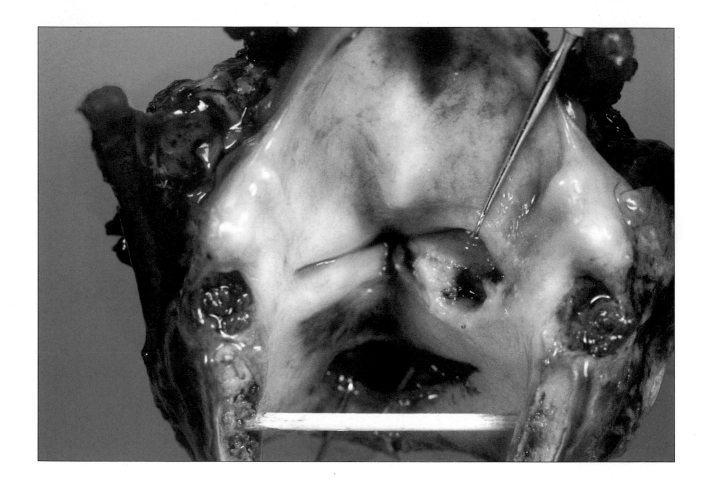

PLATE 16. Total laryngectomy specimen for right fixed cord lesion. Initial transverse incision at cricothyroid membrane was made to determine suitability for hemilaryngectomy. Submucosal induration indicated that the inferior margin would have been too close to the tumor. (Reprinted from Kirchner JA, Carter D. The Larynx. In: Sternberg SS, ed. *Diagnostic Surgical Pathology* 2nd ed [Fig 19]. New York: Raven Press, © 1994, with permission.)

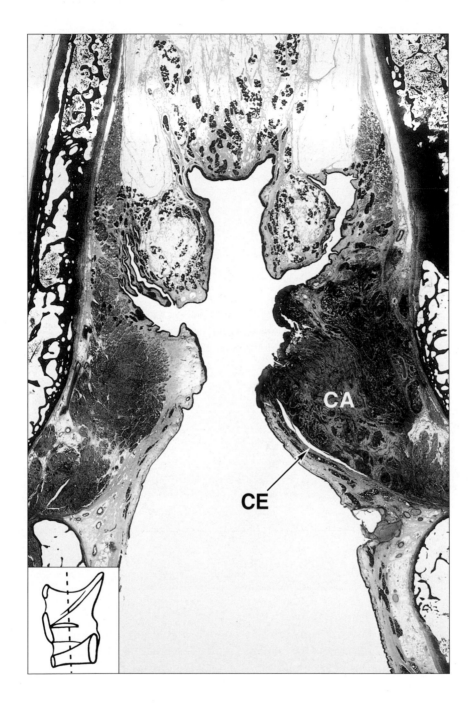

PLATE 17. Coronal section, mid-larynx, of the previous specimen showing tumor extending inferiorly under conus elasticus (CE). The tumor (CA) has invaded the free edge of the true cord and destroyed most of the thyroarytenoid muscle. Below the point of invasion, the tumor is contained within the space bounded medially by the conus elasticus (CE). Submucosal separation of tumor from the overlying mucosa during fixation shows that the lower part of the conus is still intact. (Reprinted from Kirchner JA. Spread and Barriers to Spread of Cancer within the Larynx. In: Silver CE, ed. *Laryngeal Cancer* [Fig 2-4]. New York: Thieme, © 1991, with permission.)

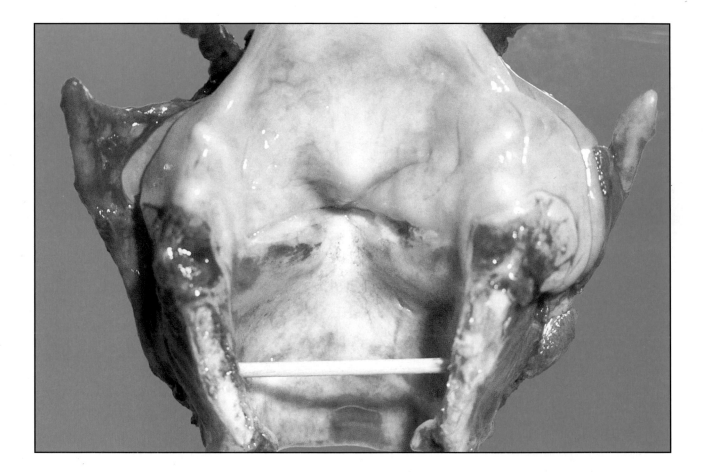

PLATE 18. Total laryngectomy for right glottic carcinoma, mainly submucosal. Full-course irradiation (6700r) had been delivered 13 months before the opera- tion. Palpable induration was now present below the glottic level, with a small tumor visible at the posterior end of the true cord.

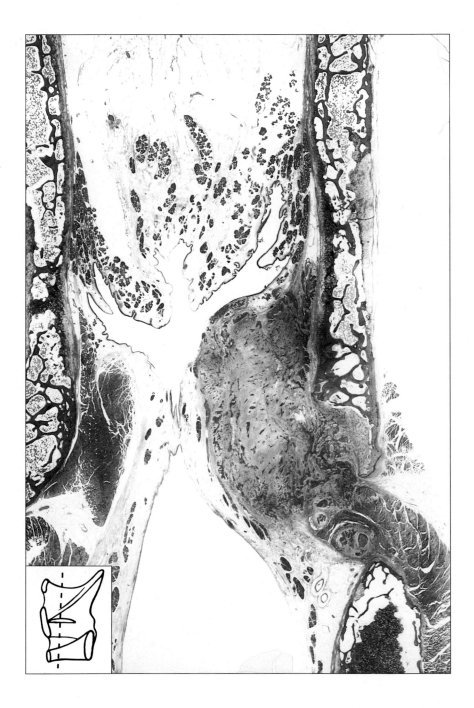

PLATE 19. Coronal section showing tumor having replaced the thyroarytenoid muscle, invaded the lower edge of the thyroid cartilage (arrow) and escaped through the cricothyroid membrane. Mucosal surface is largely intact, possibly having healed during radiotherapy. (Reprinted from Kirchner JA. Spread and Barriers to Spread of Cancer within the Larynx. In: Silver CE, ed. *Laryngeal Cancer* [Fig 2-5]. New York: Thieme, © 1991, with permission.)

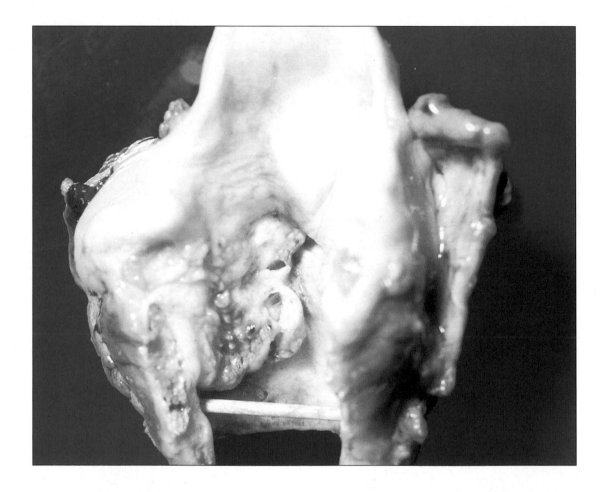

PLATE 20. Glottic carcinoma with more than 1-cm extension below the glottic level. It had been treated, unsuccessfully, with full-course irradiation.

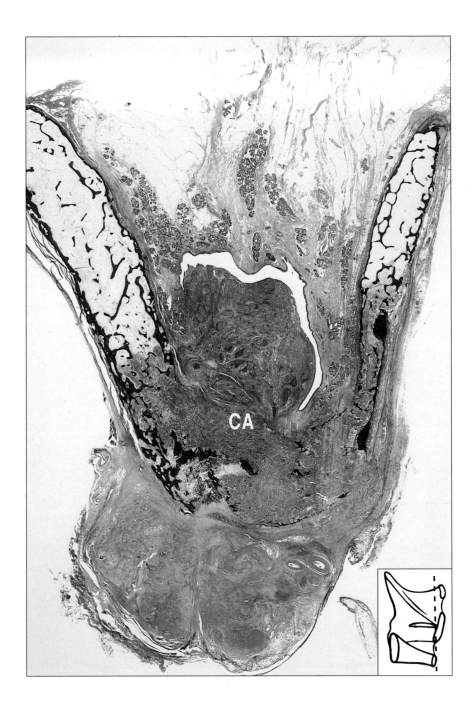

PLATE 21. Coronal section of the previous specimen (CA) through the anterior larynx. Subglottic exten-sion of tumor has destroyed the lower part of the thy-roid lamina and invaded the cricothyroid space.

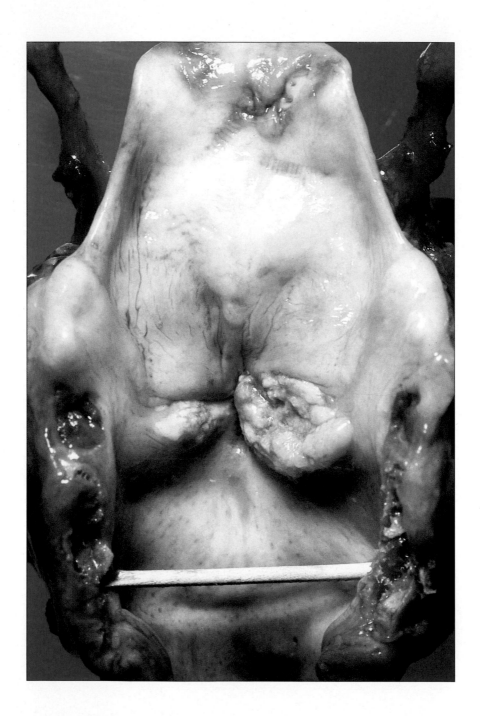

PLATE 22. Right glottic carcinoma with fixed vocal cord. The subglottic part of the lesion does not extend more than 1 cm and could have been managed by hemi-laryngectomy. The operation was considered inadvisable because of dysplastic changes on the left cord.

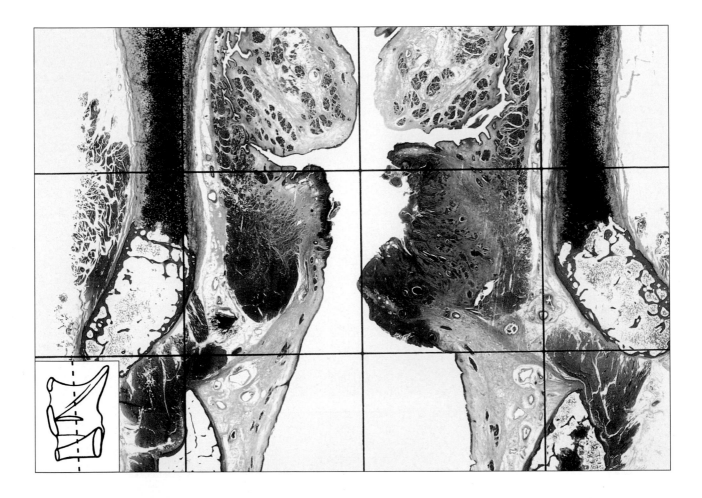

PLATE 23. Coronal section, total laryngectomy, 1-cm grid. The lower edge of tumor does not extend to the top of the cricoid. The opposite cord shows dysplastic changes. This type of lesion, or bilateral glottic cancer, could be controlled by supracricoid laryngectomy.[6] (Reprinted from Kirchner JA, Carter D. The Larynx. In: Sternberg SS, ed. *Diagnostic Surgical Pathology* 2nd ed [Fig 18]. New York: Raven Press, © 1994, with permission.)

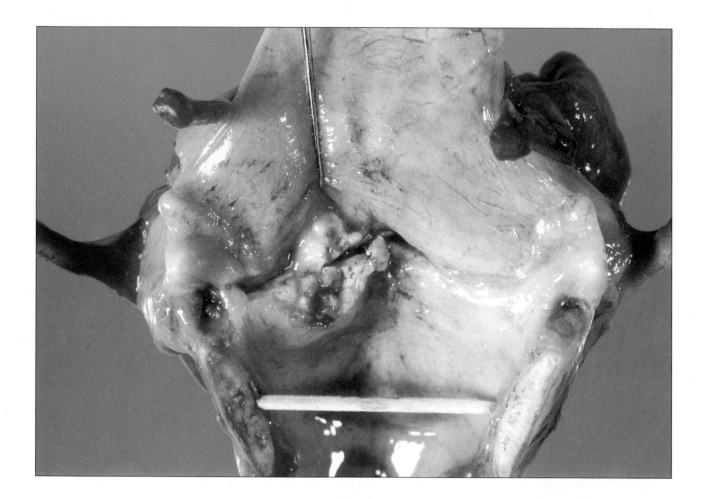

PLATE 24. Indurated, fixed left true cord with smooth, intact mucosal surface below visible tumor. The extent of tumor on the floor of the ventricle could not be determined on indirect laryngoscopy. The lower part of the false cord was displaced upward, but not indurated.

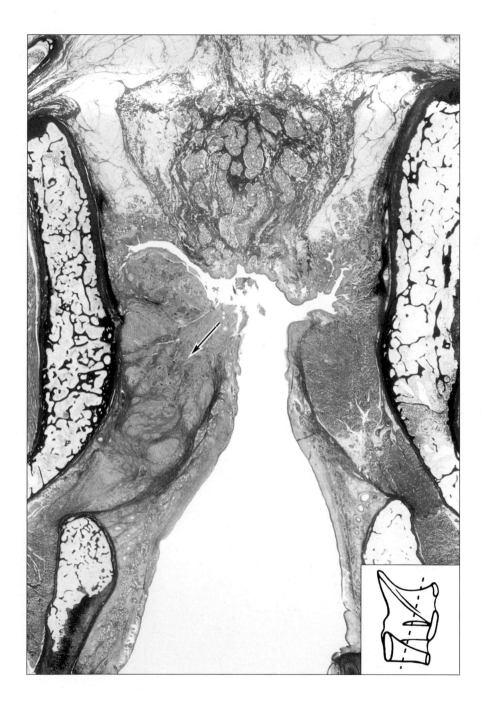

PLATE 25. Coronal section, elastic tissue stain. Carcinoma has broken through the vocal ligament near its free edge (arrow) and invaded the thyroarytenoid mus-cle. Tumor occupies the floor of the ventricle but has not crossed the fundus.

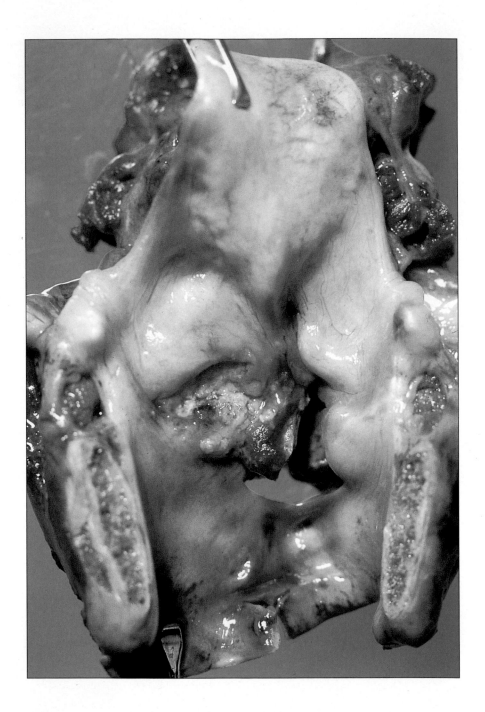

PLATE 26. Preoperatively, the left false cord appeared swollen and indurated. The glottic portion of the tumor could not be seen at indirect laryngoscopy. The initial transverse incision in the cricothyroid membrane was made to evaluate the lesion for hemilaryngectomy.

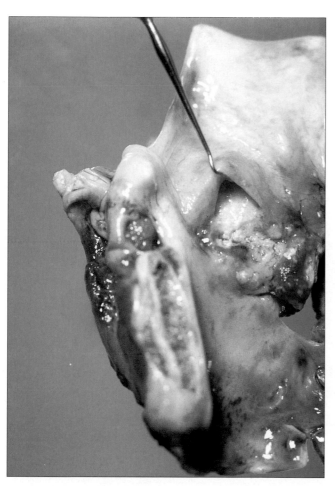

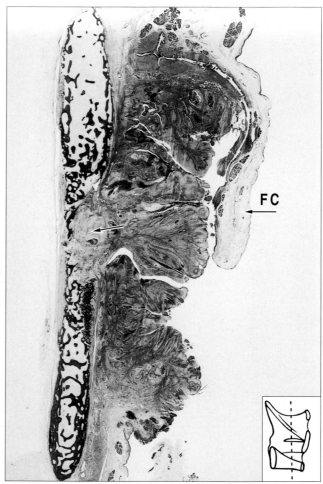

PLATE 27. The glottic tumor in the previous plate extends upward under an intact false cord.

PLATE 28. Coronal section of the laryngectomy specimen. Glottic carcinoma has extended upward into a large ventricle or internal laryngocele under an intact false cord (FC). Unlike carcinoma originating on the false cord itself, this lesion has invaded the thyroid lamina (arrow) and burrowed under the quadrangular membrane.

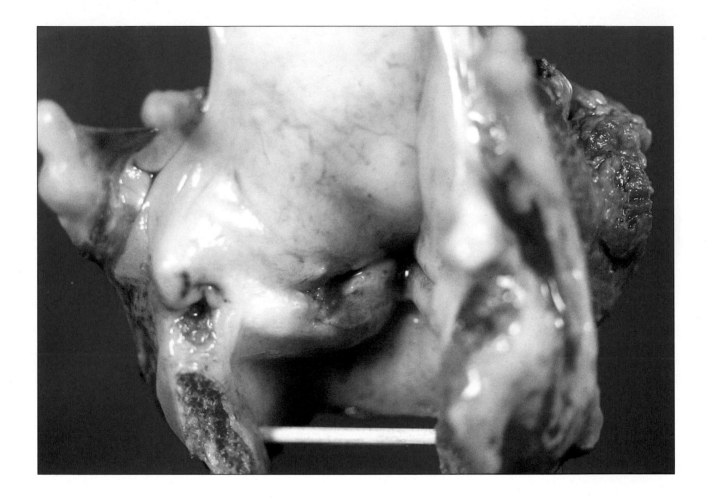

PLATE 29. Left glottic cancer, recurrent 3 years after radiotherapy. When irradiation fails to cure glottic cancer, it may allow the surface to heal while the submucosal tumor remains. The only evidence of recurrent tumor in this case was a fixed, indurated cord without visible tumor. The defect in the left true cord occurred at biopsy.

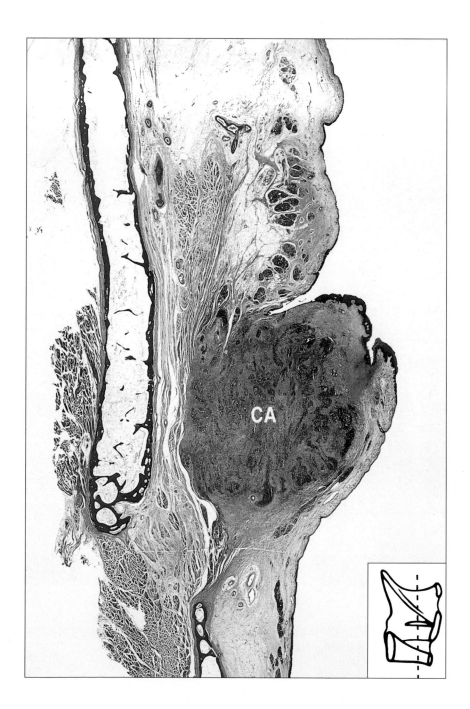

PLATE 30. Coronal section through left side of the previous specimen. Surface mucosa is thickened but intact. Tumor (CA) has replaced most of the glottic musculature. A biopsy attempt after radiotherapy often fails to reach the tumor, and the resulting break in the surface mucosa heals slowly, if at all.

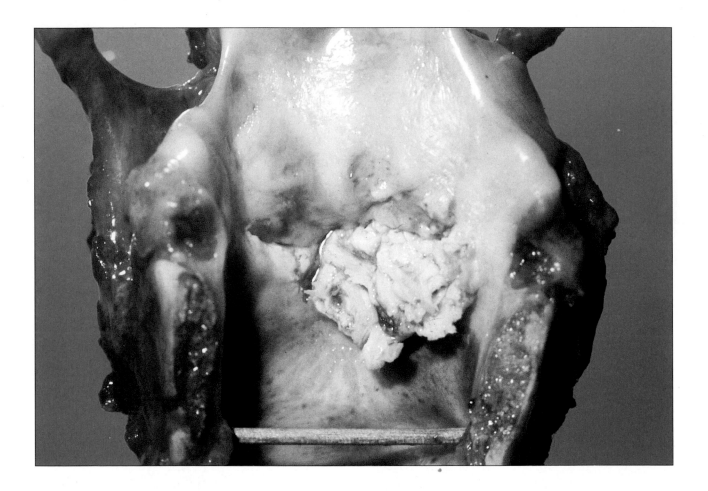

PLATE 31. Verrucous carcinoma, both true cords. Verrucous lesions in our experience did not invade deeply and often were amenable to laser resection or conservation surgery.[7]

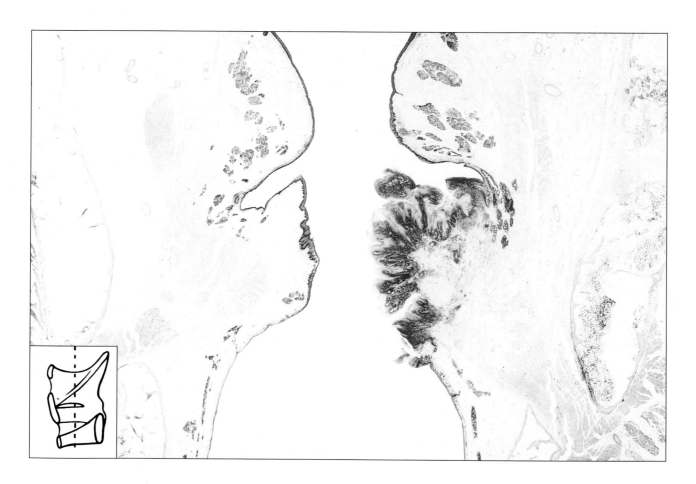

PLATE 32. Coronal section of the previous lesion showing minimal invasion.

REFERENCES

1. Kirchner JA. Invasion of the framework by laryngeal cancer. *Acta Otolaryngol (Stockh).* 1984;97:392–397.
2. Friedrich G. Surgical Anatomy of the Larynx. In: Kleinsasser O, Glanz H, Olofsson J, eds. *Advances in Laryngology in Europe.* Amsterdam: Elsevier; 1997; 337–341.
3. Som ML. Cordal cancer with extension to vocal process. *Laryngoscope.* 1975;85:1298–1307.
4. Laccourreye O, Ross J, Brasnu D, Chabardes E, Kelly JH, Laccourreye H. Extended supracricoid partial laryngectomy with tracheocricohyoidoepiglottopexy. *Acta Oto-Laryngol.* 1994;114(6):669–674.
5. Blaugrund S, Kurland S. Arytenoid replacement following hemilaryngectomy. *Laryngoscope.* 1975;85: 935–941.
6. deVincentiis M, Minni A, Gallo A. Supracricoid laryngectomy with cricohyoidopexy (CHP) in the treatment of laryngeal cancer: a functional and oncologic experience. *Laryngoscope.* 1996;106:1108–1114.
7. Ferlito A. Diagnosis and treatment of verrucous squamous cell carcinoma of the larynx. A critical review. *Ann Otol Rhinol Laryngol.* 1985;94:575–579.

ANTERIOR COMMISSURE CANCER

Most glottic cancer arises in the anterior cord, where lymphatics are sparse[1] and where the glottic and supraglottic vasculature is interrupted at the anterior commissure.[2] Invasion of the thyroid cartilage by cancer at the anterior commissure may be accurately predicted by its surface presentation.

A tumor crossing from one mobile cord to the other, but restricted to the level of the glottis, does not invade the thyroid cartilage. Of the 20 such specimens studied by serial section, the adjacent thyroid cartilage has not been invaded in a single instance.

Glottic cancer spreading downward from the anterior commissure has not invaded the thyroid cartilage in our specimens unless it extended to or below its lower edge, approximately 1 cm below the anterior commissure.

A tumor spreading upward from the anterior commissure rarely occurs unless it is part of a larger, fixed cord lesion. Instead, it is "stopped by the basket-like fibrous structure formed by the caudal end of Broyles ligament[3] together with the thyroid cartilage and the insertion of the vocal muscles."[4 (p308)] When invasion of the epiglottic petiole does occur, the tumor is usually ulcerated and nearly always invades the thyroid cartilage (cf. Plate #42). The difficulty of determining the vertical dimension of a tumor at the anterior commissure may account for discrepancies in reported rates of framework invasion.[5-7]

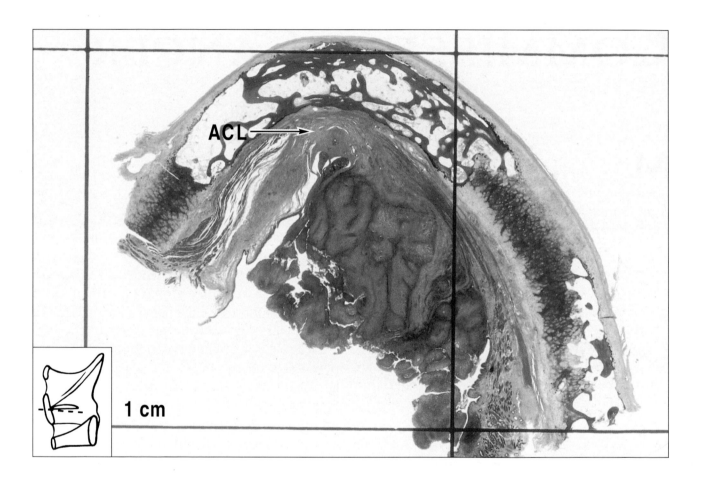

PLATE 33. Transverse section, glottic carcinoma removed by fronto-lateral resection. Tumor does not cross the commissure and is being contained at this level by the anterior commissure ligament (ACL). (Reprinted from Ariyan S. *Cancer of the Head and Neck* [Fig 15-1]. St. Louis: Mosby, © 1987, with permission.)

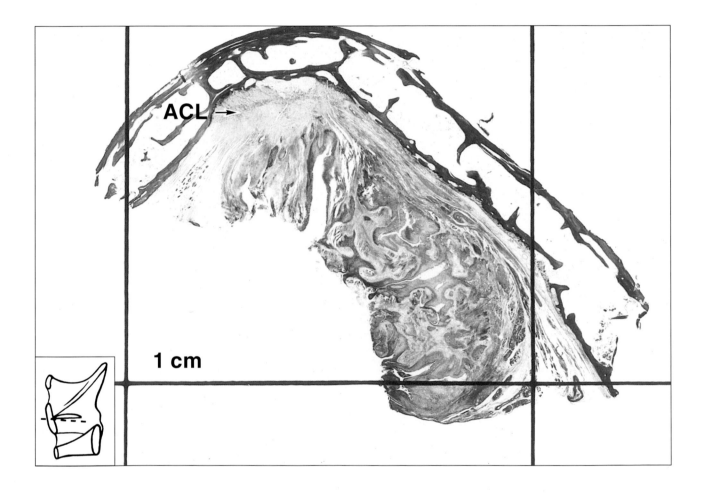

PLATE 34. Transverse section of a small fixed glottic carcinoma removed by fronto-lateral resection. Carcinoma has reached the anterior commissure, but has invaded neither the ligament (ACL) nor the thyroid cartilage.

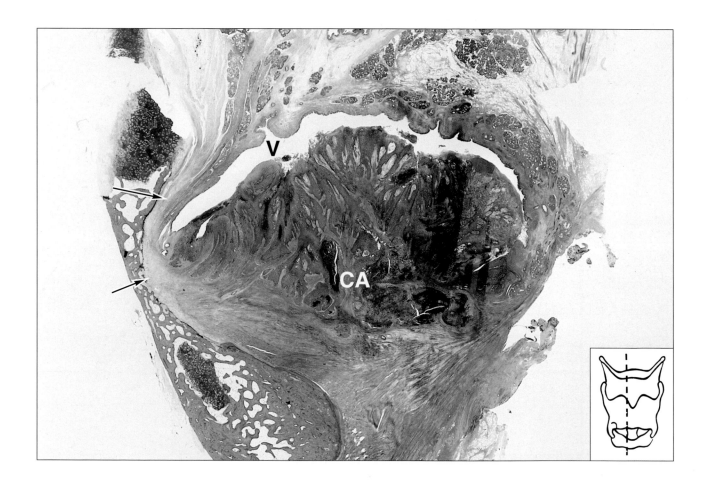

PLATE 34.1. Parasagittal section of glottic cancer showing a vertical view along Broyles ligament above, below, and just lateral to the anterior commissure (arrows). CA = cancer V = ventricle

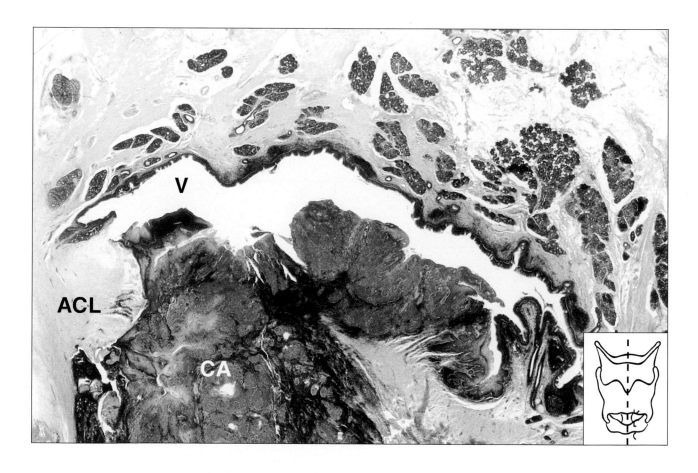

PLATE 34.2. Oblique-sagittal section of glottic cancer showing the "small fibrous projection (ACL) which serves for the insertion of the vocal cords" described by Ridpath.[8] CA = cancer V = ventricle

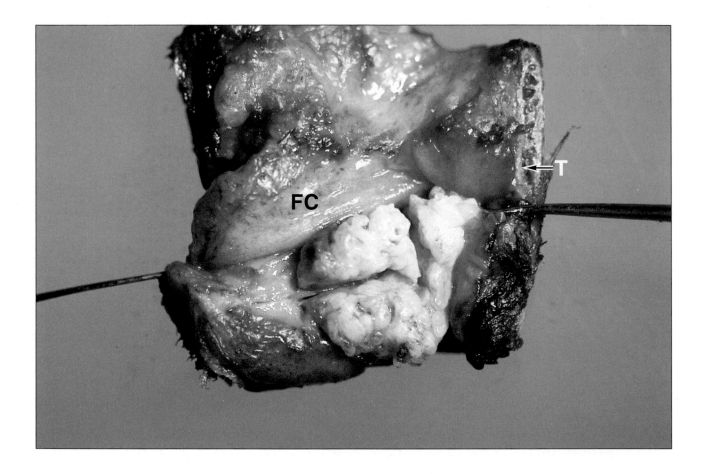

PLATE 35. This verrucous carcinoma was resected by the anterior commissure technique. A tumor at the anterior commissure may be difficult to evaluate preop- eratively for location and extent. Adequate margins are visible to the right and left of the tumor. FC = false cord T = thyroid cartilage

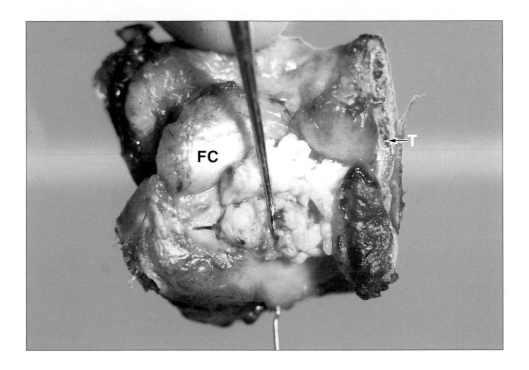

PLATE 36. The overhanging lower edge of the same tumor gave a false impression of subglottic spread, but its base is well above the lower line of resection. FC = false cord T = thyroid cartilage

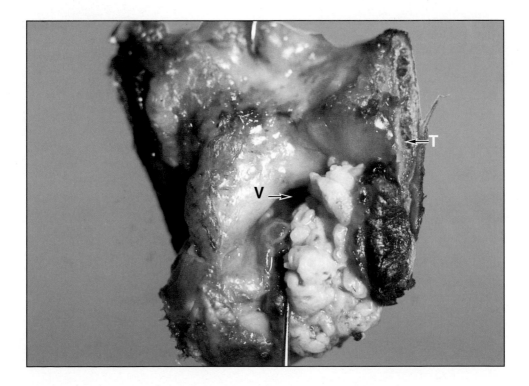

PLATE 37. Superior edge of the tumor overlies the base of the epiglottis but has not invaded it. Ventricle (V) is clear. Typically, this verrucous carcinoma showed minimal invasion of the underlying soft tissues and an intact thyroid cartilage. T = thyroid cartilage

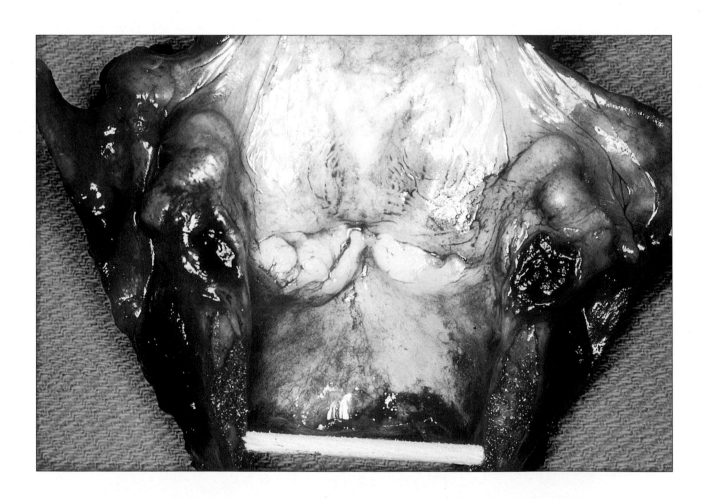

PLATE 38. Bilateral glottic carcinoma, verrucoid. With mobile vocal cords, infraglottic spread limited to a few millimeters and the base of the epiglottis free of vis- ible tumor, the thyroid cartilage is invariably intact. Sections are unavailable for this lesion, but a more advanced lesion is shown in the following section.

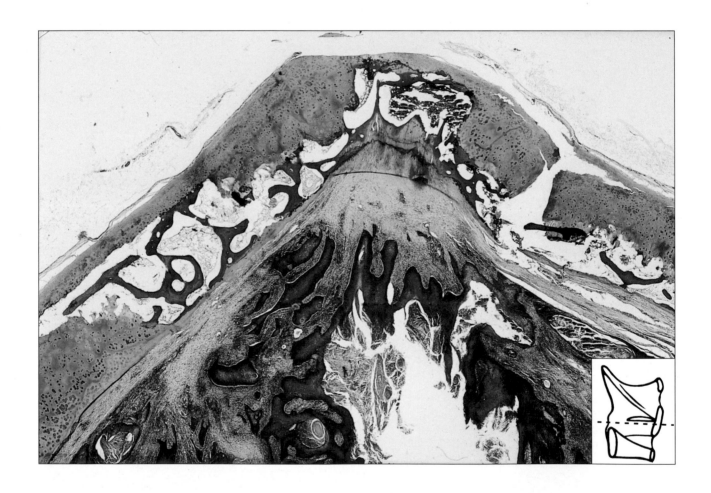

PLATE 39. Bilateral, fixed cord lesion. Despite its bilaterality and large size, it has not invaded the anterior commissure tendon. The fracture to the right of the mid- line results when the laryngectomy specimen is spread open to inspect the tumor.

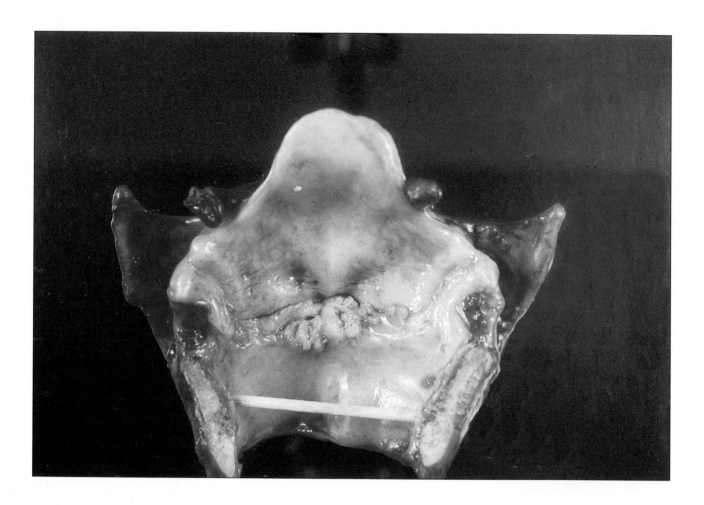

PLATE 40. Glottic carcinoma limited to a few millimeters extension below the glottis. The base of the epiglottis is free of visible tumor. Framework invasion is unlikely.

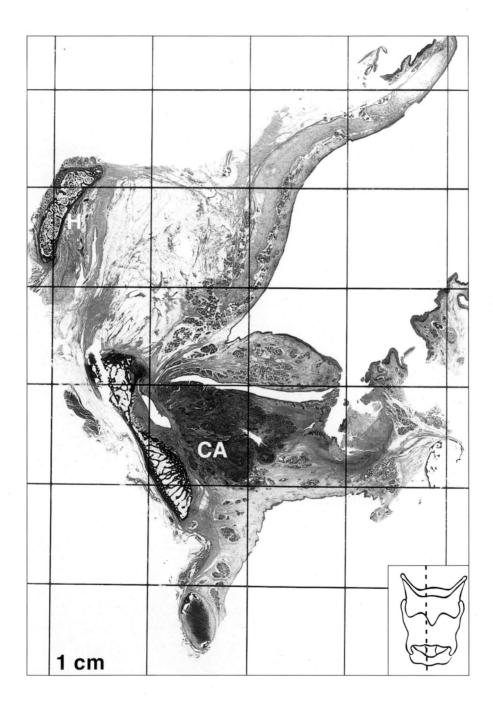

1 cm

PLATE 41. Parasagittal section of the previous specimen. The tumor spreads less than 1 cm below the glottic level and has not invaded the adjacent framework. CA = cancer

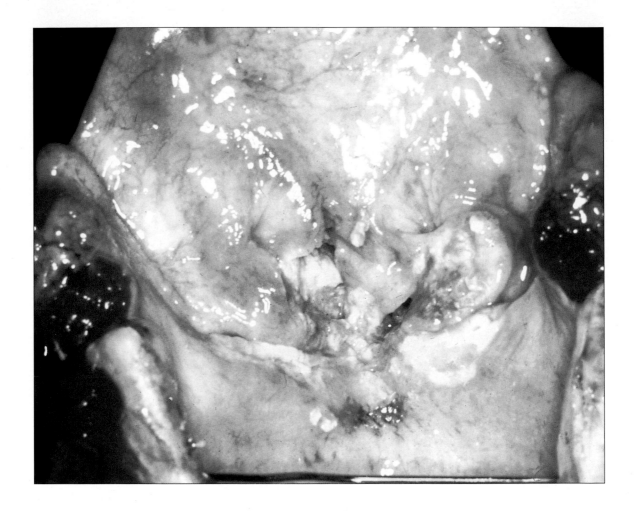

PLATE 42. Carcinoma rarely crosses the anterior commissure in a vertical direction, whether its origin is glottic or supraglottic. When it does, it is invariably part of a much more extensive tumor involving other parts of the larynx. Such lesions usually invade the adjacent laryngeal framework (13 of 17 nonirradiated surgical specimens studied).[9] (Reprinted from Kirchner JA. The Systems of UICC and AJC for Staging of Laryngeal Carcinoma. In: Wigand ME, Steiner W, Stell PM, eds. *Functional Partial Laryngectomy* [Fig 1, p 70]. New York: Springer-Verlag, © 1984, with permission.)

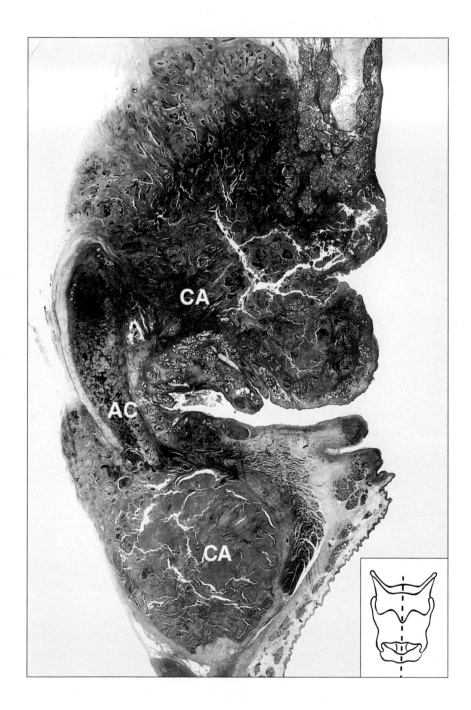

PLATE 43. Midsagittal section of previous specimen. Cancer (CA) above and below the anterior commissure (AC) has invaded and destroyed the lower part of the thyroid cartilage. Below the true cord, cancer (CA) is present in the framework.

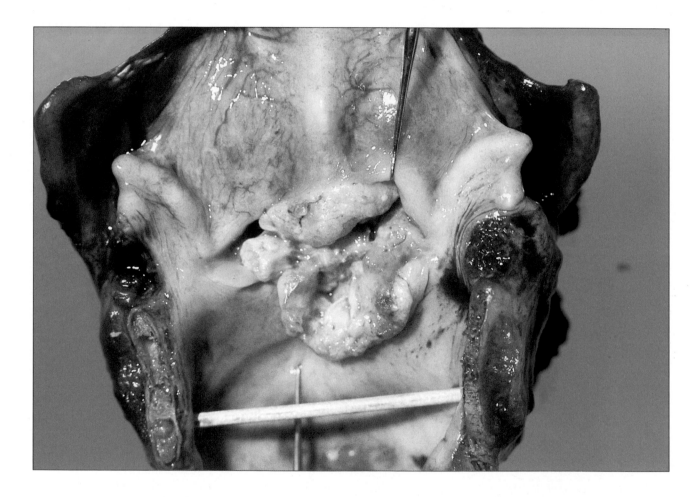

PLATE 44. Glottic carcinoma extending upward to the base of the epiglottis. Despite its exophytic appearance, its position above and below the anterior commissure predicts invasion of the adjacent framework.

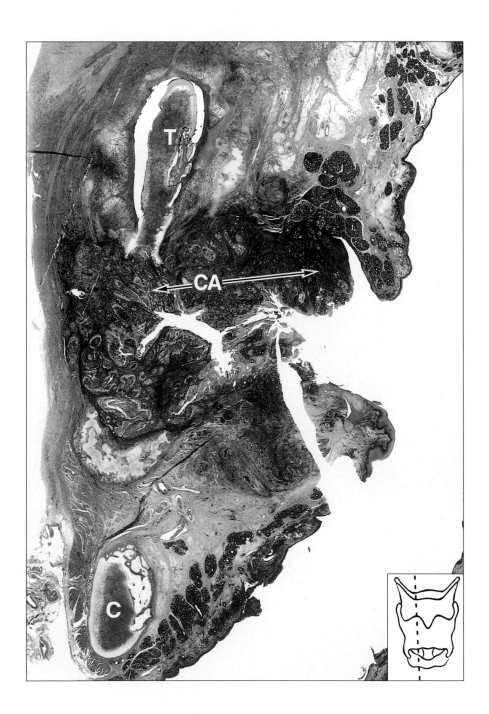

PLATE 45. Parasagittal section of the previous specimen shows extensive destruction of the anterior part of the thyroid cartilage. Lesions of this type are classified "transglottic" in our practice. T = thyroid cartilage CA = cancer C = cricoid cartilage

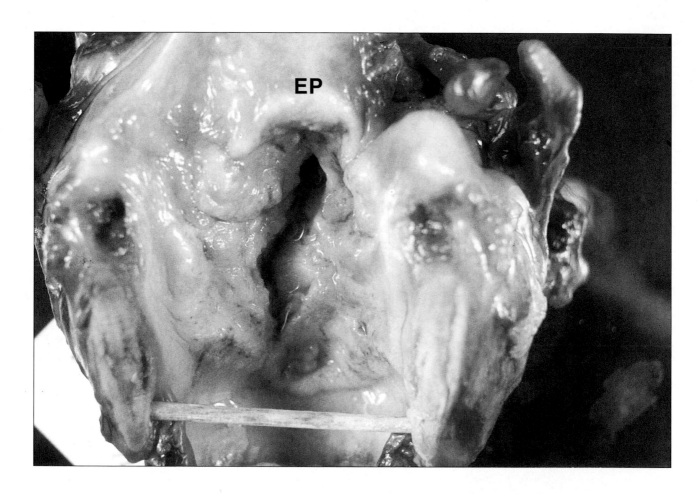

PLATE 46. A deeply ulcerated type of lesion above and below the anterior commissure. EP = base of epiglottis

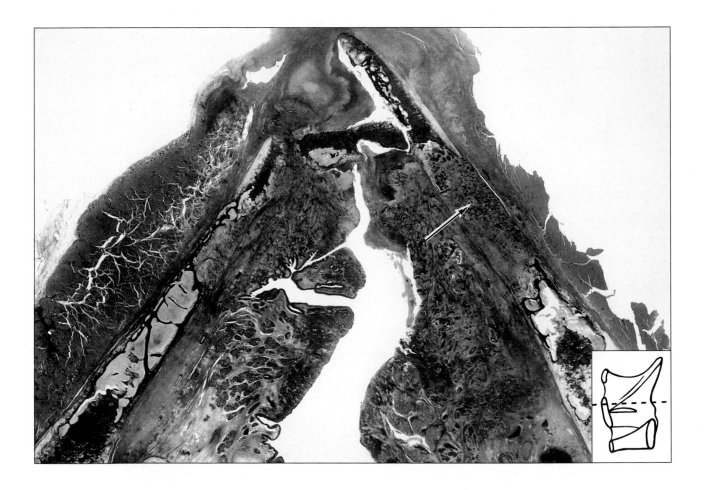

PLATE 47. Transverse section of the previous specimen showing invasion of the thyroid lamina (arrow) and destruction of the framework at the anterior part of the larynx. Fragments of unossified cartilage remain.

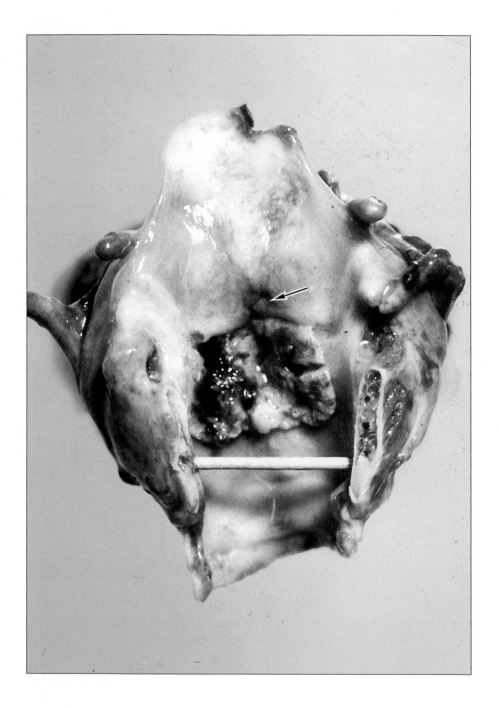

PLATE 48. This surgical specimen illustrates the difficulty in assessing the base of the epiglottis without telescopic equipment. The swelling above the anterior commissure (arrow) was caused by submucosal extension of visible tumor. Inferior extension of the tumor exceeds 1 cm, an additional indication of framework invasion.

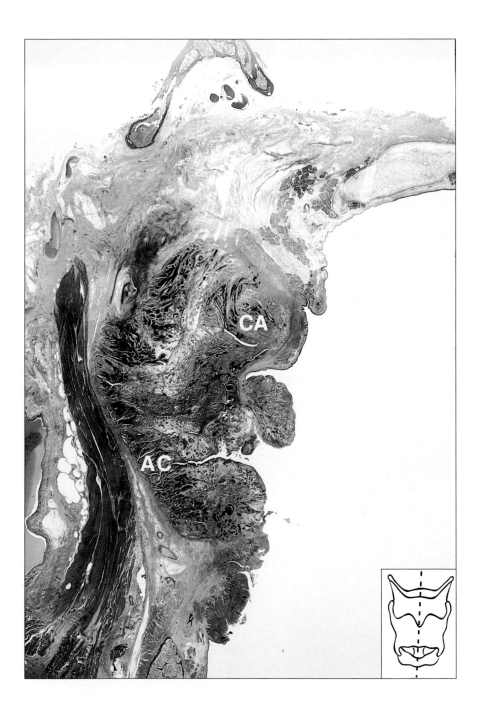

PLATE 49. Midsagittal section of the previous specimen. Submucosal tumor (CA) is seen just above the base of the epiglottis. Carcinoma has invaded and destroyed most of the thyroid cartilage above and below the anterior commissure (AC). A portion of the sternohyoid muscle is seen on the left.

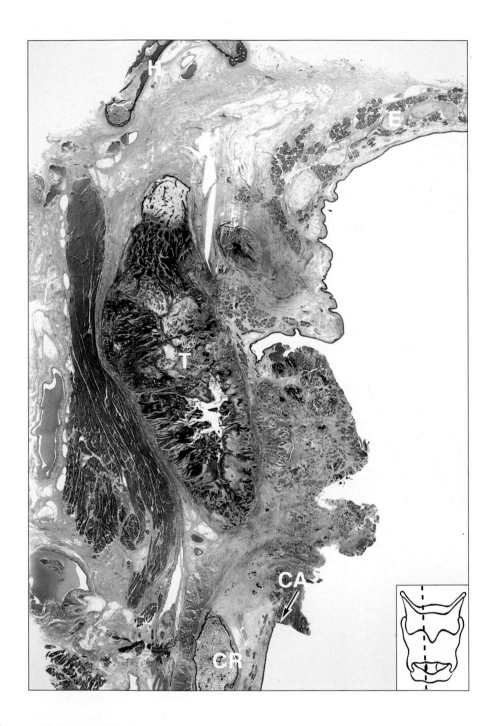

PLATE 50. Parasagittal section of the same specimen. Tumor (CA) has extended more than 1 cm below the anterior commissure and invaded the thyroid cartilage (T). The lower margin of visible tumor is seen at the arrow. CR = cricoid H = hyoid bone E = epiglottis

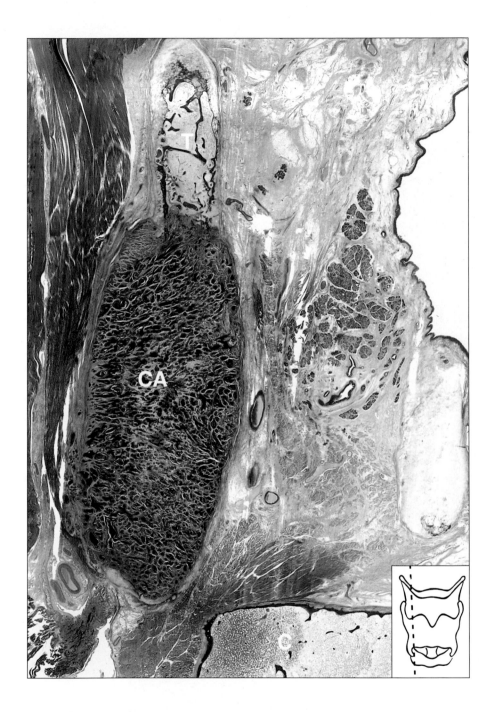

PLATE 51. Parasagittal section of the previous specimen, more lateral. Carcinoma within the thyroid cartilage expands the lamina between internal and external layers of perichondrium. Overlying soft tissue shows no evidence of tumor at this plane. T = thyroid cartilage CA = cancer C = cricoid cartilage

REFERENCES

1. Werner JA, Schünke M, Rudert H, Tillman B. Description and clinical importance of the lymphatics of the vocal fold. *Otolaryngology-Head and Neck Surgery.* 1990;102:13–19.
2. Andrea M. (1981). Vasculature of the anterior commissure. *Ann Otol Rhinol Laryngol.* 1981;90(pt 1): 18–20.
3. Broyles EN. The anterior commissure tendon. *Ann. Otol.* 1943;52:342–345.
4. Rucci L, Gammarota L, Cirri, MBB. Carcinoma of the anterior commissure of the larynx: 1. Embryological and anatomic considerations. *Ann Otol Rhinol Laryngol.* 1996;105(4):303–308.
5. Bagatella F, Bignardi L. Behavior of cancer at the anterior commissure of the larynx. *Laryngoscope.* 1983; 93:353–356.
6. Olofsson J. Specific features of laryngeal carcinoma involving the anterior commissure and subglottic region. In: Alberti WP, Bryce DW, eds. *Workshops from the Centennial Conference on Laryngeal Cancer.* New York: Appleton-Century-Crofts; 1976;626–644.
7. Rucci L, Gammarota L, Gallo O. Carcinoma of the anterior commissure of the larynx: II. Proposal of a new staging system. *Ann Otol Rhinol Laryngol.* 1996; 105(5):391–396.
8. Ridpath RF. Anatomy of the larynx. In: *The Nose, Throat and Ear, and Their Diseases.* Jackson and Coates, Philadelphia and London, W.B. Saunders Co. 1929: 737, (cited by Broyles).
9. Kirchner JA. "What have whole organ sections contributed to the treatment of laryngeal cancer?" *Ann Otol Rhinol Laryngol.* 1989;98:661–667.

TRANSGLOTTIC CANCER

The term "transglottic" was introduced in a report by McGavran et al in 1961[1] as a definition of a tumor's location rather than a supposition as to where it began. The term is clinically useful, although imprecise, because it denotes cancer with a surface presentation both above and below the entrance to the ventricle, rather than above and below the glottis. A glottic tumor, for example, spreading upward into a large ventricle under an intact false cord would not qualify as "transglottic" even though its superior edge is well above the level of the glottis. A serpiginous lesion on the glottic and supraglottic mucosa would be termed "transglottic" in some practices, but would require a fixed true cord in others. In this series the term "transglottic" was assigned to those lesions with surface presentation both above and below the entrance to the ventricle or anterior commissure, with a fixed true vocal cord. Regardless of its point of origin, the location of a visible tumor on the glottic and/or supraglottic components of the larynx and the tumor's size are what determine, in large part, the likelihood of invasion of the laryngeal framework and of cervical node metastasis.

Of 91 transglottic tumors studied by whole-organ section, 46 (51%) showed invasion of the thyroid and/or cricoid cartilages. Cervical node metastasis from transglottic cancer showed a direct relation to the size of the primary lesion in our specimens. Among the 39 lesions under 4 cm, regional metastases appeared in 9 cases (23%), whereas 11 lesions over 4 cm produced metastases in 6 (55%).[2] Glottic carcinoma may spread posteriorly behind the ventricle and upward onto the false cord. This is the usual route of the lesion that becomes transglottic, encircling the ventricle before obliterating it.[3]

In a much less common form, the tumor may involve the true cord, false cord, ventricle, base of the epiglottis and/or anterior commissure, with the retro-ventricular portion of the tumor relatively unimpressive on inspection. Its site of origin is usually impossible to determine (cf. Plate 56).

A tumor may arise on the true cord and spread upward into the ventricle or a laryngocele. The overlying false cord in this case is intact, and appears to be swollen, but indurated. It is not termed "transglottic" in our practice, because the overlying mucosa of the false cord shows no carcinoma (cf. Plate 26).

Submucosal cancer observed above and below the ventricle in whole-organ sections may have originated in the pyriform sinus, whose anterior edge lies in contact with the paraglottic space. Once established within this space, cancer can spread, submucosally, above and below the ventricular fundus, but not be classifiable as transglottic.

Examples of various patterns of invasion are shown in the following specimens.

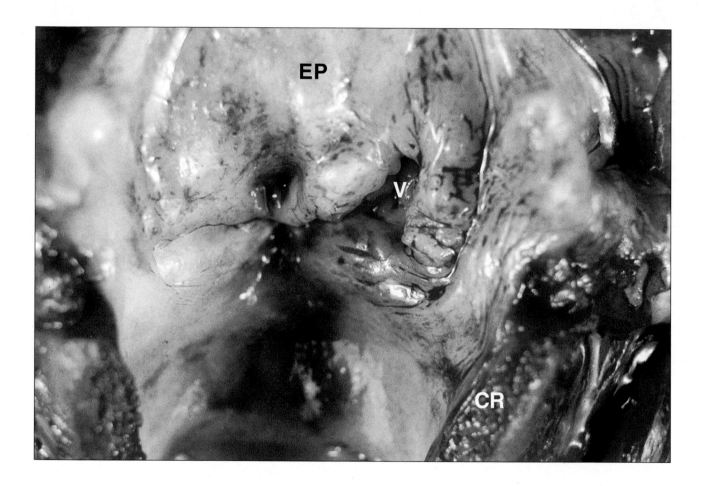

PLATE 52. Total laryngectomy specimen with a tumor on the right true cord, false cord, and behind the ventricle (V), illustrating an early stage of transglottic carcinoma. The ventricle is still identifiable and has not yet been obliterated. EP = epiglottis CR = cricoid

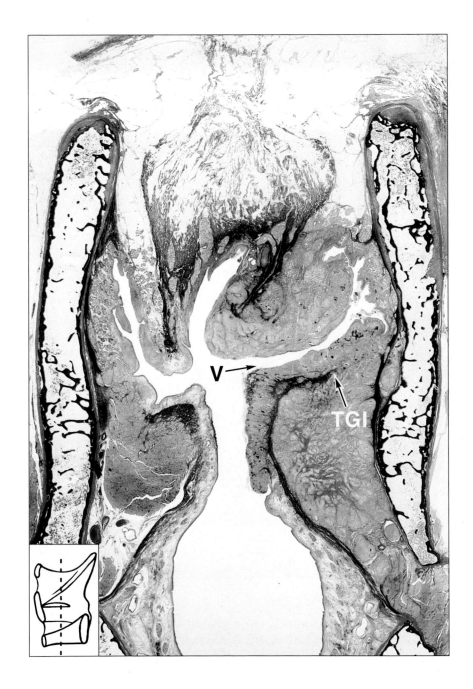

PLATE 53. Coronal section, elastic tissue stain of the previous specimen. The thyroglottic ligament (TGl) is incomplete, suggesting that carcinoma originating on the true cord may have out-flanked the ligament, invaded the thyroarytenoid muscle below and the supra-glottic area above. The persistence of the ventricular cleft (V), however, provides strong evidence that the tumor has "surrounded" the ventricle from behind, invading both the glottic and supraglottic parts of the larynx. The ventricle has not been "crossed" but encircled.[3]

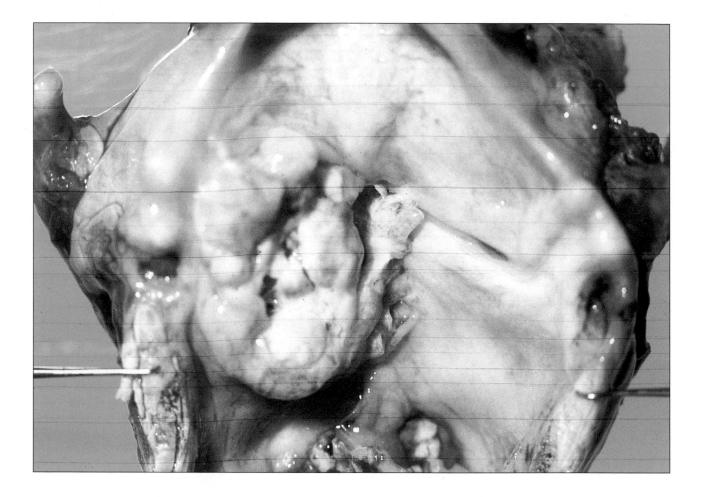

PLATE 54. In this total laryngectomy specimen, the tumor has surrounded the left ventricle from behind and invaded both the true and false cords. This type of lesion is associated with a fixed true cord and is deeply invasive. Visible and palpable tumor measures nearly 4 cm, a useful dimension when predicting framework invasion in transglottic cancer.[2] (Reprinted from Kirchner JA, Carter D. The Larynx. In: Sternberg SS, ed. *Diagnostic Surgical Pathology* 2nd ed [Fig 25]. New York: Raven Press, © 1994, with permission.)

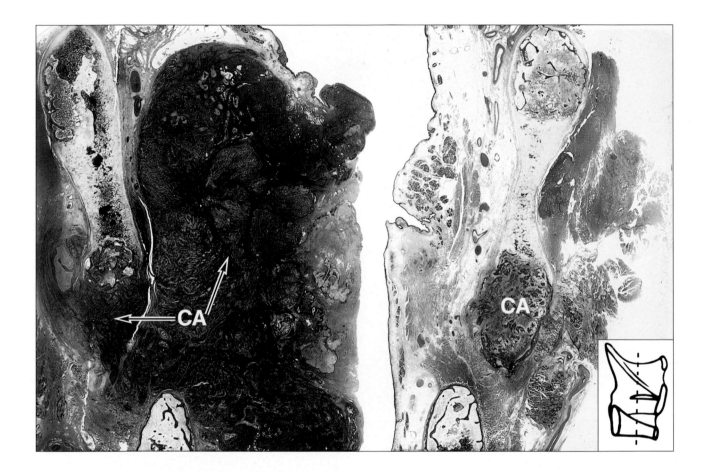

PLATE 55. Coronal section of the previous specimen. The tumor has obliterated the ventricle and invaded the lower, ossified part of the thyroid lamina (arrows). What is more important is that the tumor (CA) has spread within the framework under normal soft tissue to the opposite side. In so doing, cancer has replaced the cancellous framework between the internal and external perichondrial layers. Such infiltration has been observed only in those tumors that have destroyed the anterior thyroid cartilage. This alone would disqualify the lesion for conservation surgery. (Reprinted from Kirchner JA. Staging in Cancer of the Larynx. In: *Otolaryngology* Vol 5 [Ch 35, Fig 8]. Philadelphia: Lippincott-Raven, © 1979, with permission.)

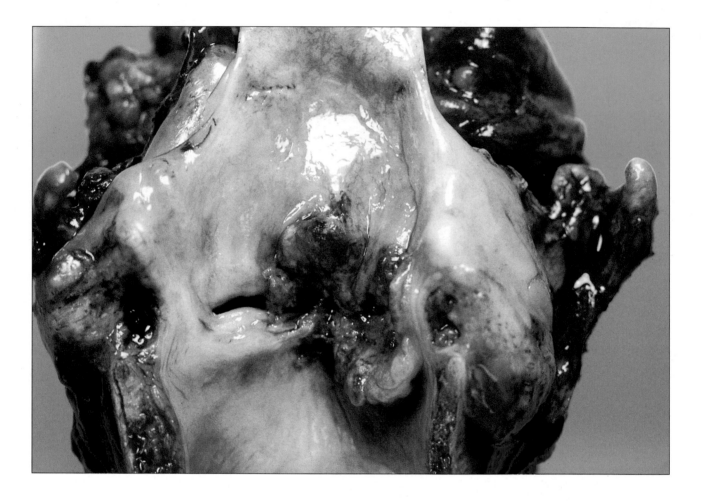

PLATE 56. This tumor occupies both the glottic and supraglottic areas, above and below both the right ventricle and the anterior commissure. The specimen illustrates the difficulty of determining the origin of this type of transglottic tumor, although gross tumor behind the ventricle suggests that the lesion, whether glottic or supraglottic in origin, may have surrounded the ventricle before obliterating it. The left true cord was mobile.

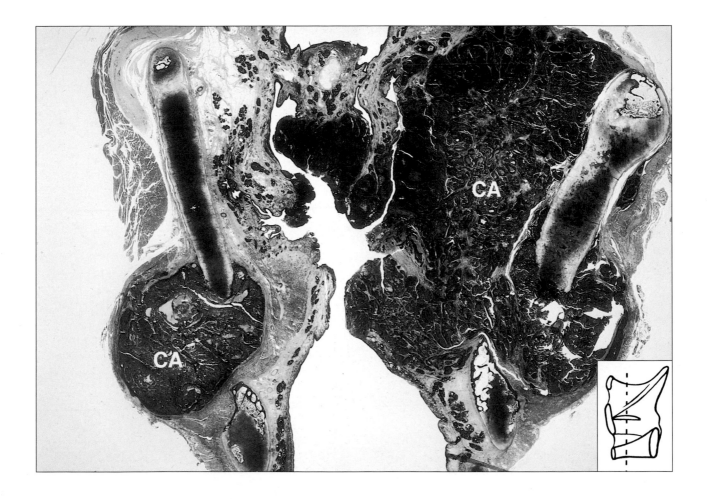

PLATE 57. Coronal section of the previous tumor. Carcinoma invades the right hemilarynx and lower edge of the thyroid ala. Additionally, the tumor has infiltrated and expanded the lower, ossified edge of the ala on the side opposite visible tumor (CA) under normal soft tissues.

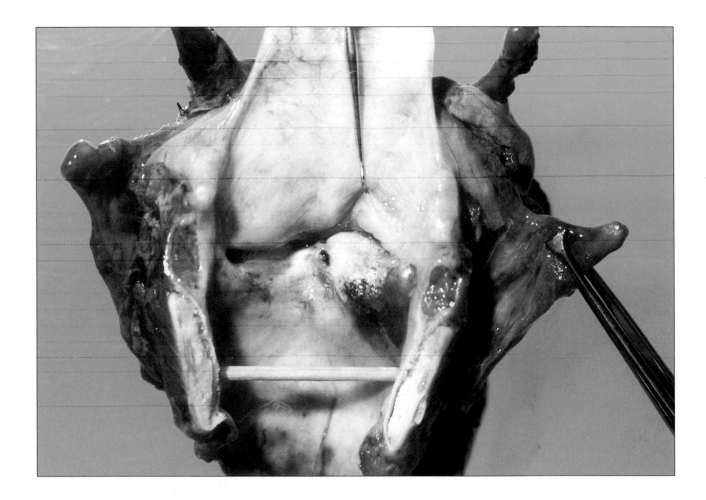

PLATE 58. Fixed right cord lesion. Upward traction by a hook reveals that the tumor extends above the fundus of the ventricle, spreading under the false cord. This is not a "transglottic" lesion in our practice. The patient had been hoarse 11 months.

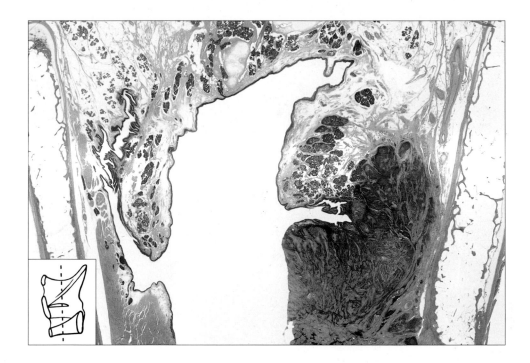

PLATE 59. Coronal section of the previous specimen. The lesion extends upward under the false cord, spreading into the right ventricle. (Compare the size of the left ventricle.) The paraglottic space has been compressed but not invaded.

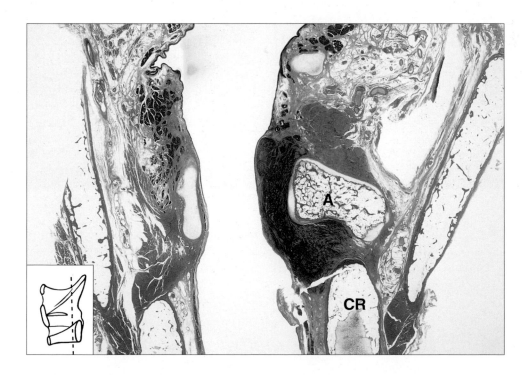

PLATE 60. In a more posterior section, the retroventricular portion of the tumor abuts the arytenoid area where it was recognizable clinically. Hemilaryngectomy for this lesion would have required resection of the arytenoid cartilage and the upper edge of the cricoid plate. This lesion was not a candidate for conventional supracricoid laryngectomy.[4] A = arytenoid cartilage CR = cricoid cartilage

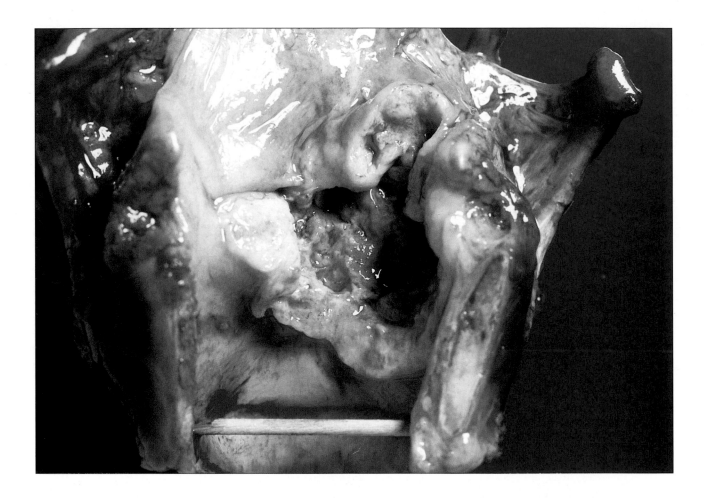

PLATE 61. The right hemilarynx is largely destroyed by what appears to have been principally a glottic-subglottic lesion. The tumor has spread to the false cord from the retroventricular area. The gross tumor measures more than 4 cm, a dimension usually indicating framework invasion in transglottic carcinoma.

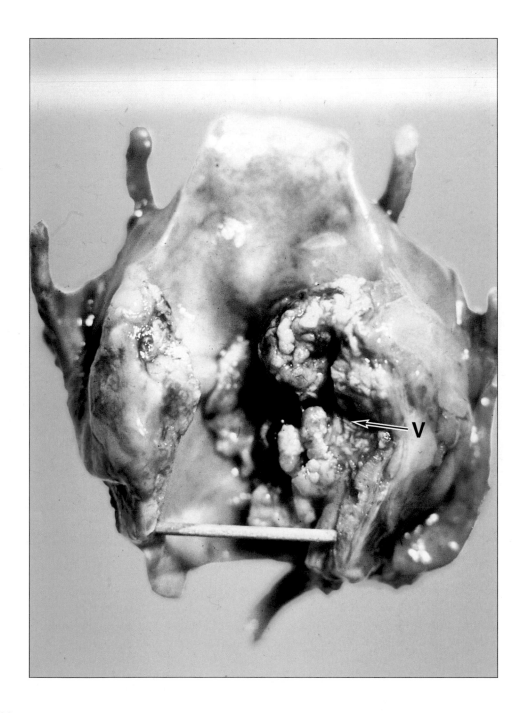

PLATE 62. In this transglottic cancer the transverse cleft within the tumor represents the remnant of the ventricle (V at arrow).

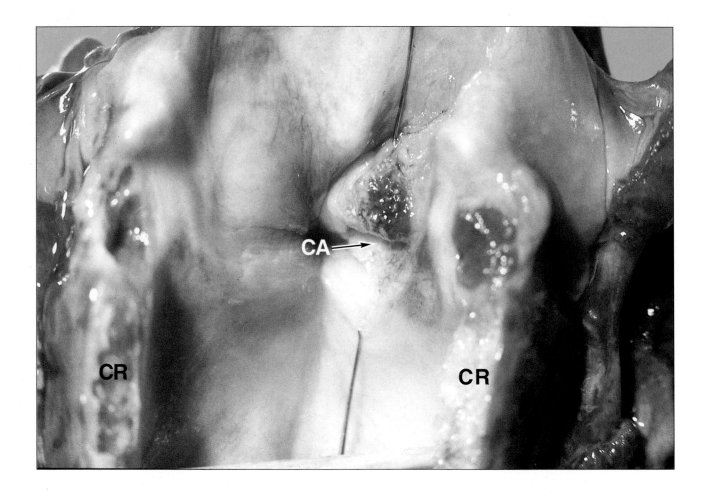

PLATE 63. Total laryngectomy specimen illustrating an entirely different pathway by which glottic cancer may spread above and below the ventricular level and not be classified "transglottic." Hooks in the true and false cords expose carcinoma (CA) deep within the ventricle at the arrow. The only evidence of tumor was indurated swelling in the right ventricular band and a fixed true cord. Several direct laryngoscopies with biopsy had failed to identify the tumor. CR = cricoid (Reprinted from Kirchner JA. Staging in Cancer of the Larynx. In: *Otolaryngology* Vol 5 [Ch 35, Fig 5]. Philadelphia: Lippincott-Raven, © 1979, with permission.)

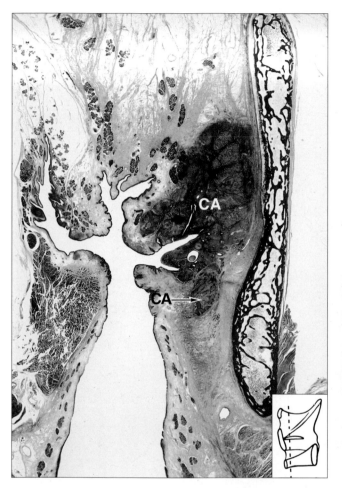

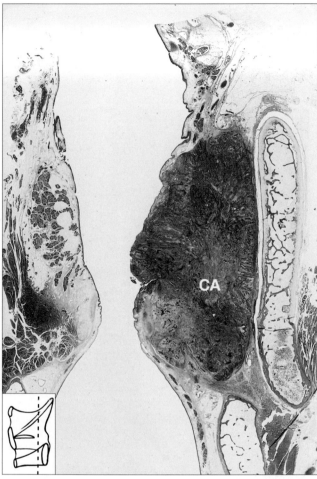

PLATE 64. Coronal section of the previous specimen. Carcinoma (CA) is deep within the ventricle, covered by normal surface mucosa at this and all other planes. The tumor (CA at arrow) has extended below the glottic level, either by breaking through the lateral part of the thyroglottic ligament or by out-flanking it and spreading downward into the thyroarytenoid muscle. (Reprinted from Mancuso AA, Hanafee WN, [Contributor: JA Kirchner]. Larynx and Hypopharynx—Normal Anatomy and Methodology. *Computed Tomography of the Head & Neck* 1st ed. [Ch. 2, Fig 2.9]. Baltimore: Williams & Wilkins, © 1982, with permission.)

PLATE 65. A more posterior section at the tumor's maximum size (CA) shows that it remains submucosal. This lesion appears to have originated on the floor of the ventricle, invaded the supraglottic and glottic areas, and destroyed the thyroarytenoid muscle. Although it lies above and below the level of the glottis, it differs from the true transglottic lesion because the supraglottic mucosa shows no obvious cancer. Strictly unilateral, this lesion might have qualified for near-total[5] or supracricoid laryngectomy.[6]

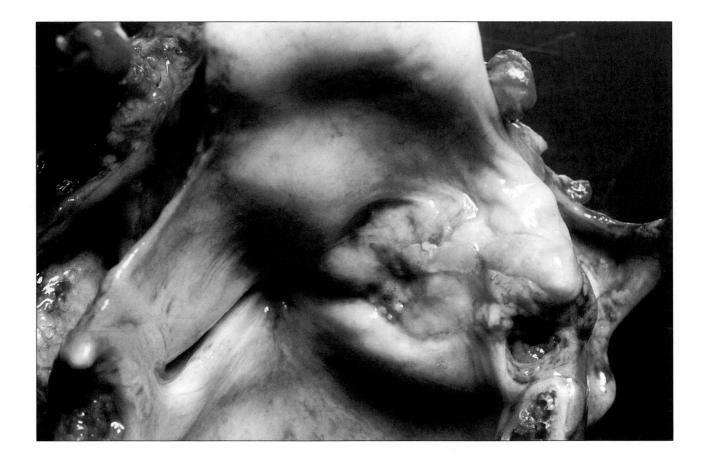

PLATE 66. This lesion began as a glottic carcinoma with fixed true cord. The tumor extended upward behind the right ventricle to the arytenoid. Because the patient refused surgery, radiotherapy was delivered, but carcinoma had spread to the false cord 2 months after irradiation and required total laryngectomy. The tumor has spread to the angle between the petiole and false cord. The right true cord is enlarged and indurated.

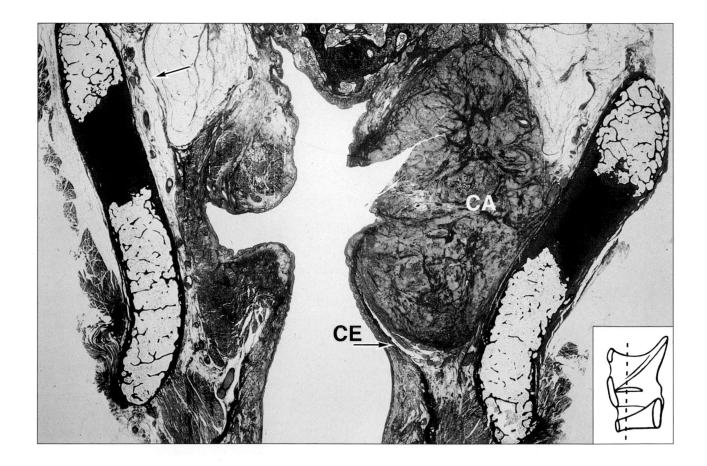

PLATE 67. Coronal section from the previous specimen. Carcinoma (CA) is seen above and below the glottis. Tumor has infiltrated the thyroarytenoid muscle deep to the conus elasticus (CE). The overlying mucosa has healed under irradiation. This specimen is a further example of how carcinoma of the true cord can extend upward behind the ventricle and eventually encircle it. On the uninvolved side, the arrow on upper left indicates the boundary between the paraglottic and preepiglottic spaces.[7]

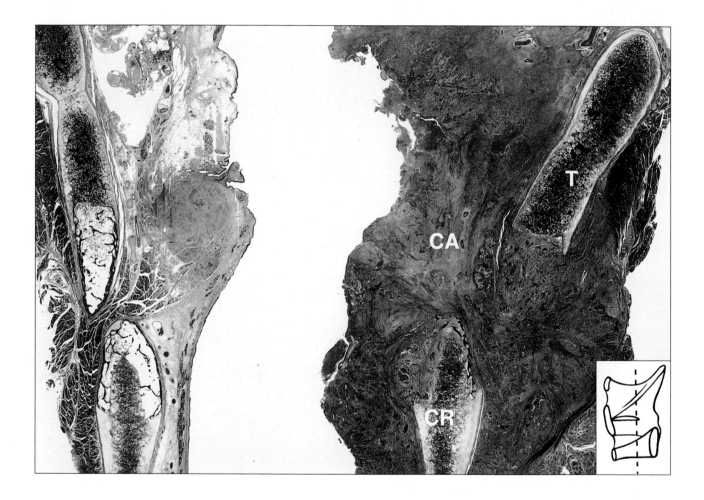

PLATE 68. Coronal section of an extensive trans-glottic carcinoma showing the preferential invasion of the ossified part of the thyroid and cricoid cartilages, primarily along muscle attachments. Unossified cartilage is still intact in this specimen. In advanced disease, the cartilage may eventually become invaded, especially in the presence of infection. T = thyroid cartilage CA = cancer CR = cricoid cartilage

REFERENCES

1. McGavran MH, Bauer WC, Ogura JH. The incidence of cervical lymph node metastases from epidermoid carcinoma of the larynx and their relationship to certain characteristics of the primary tumor. *Cancer.* 1961;14:55–66.

2. Kirchner JA, Cornog JL, Holmes RE. Transglottic cancer. *Arch Otolaryngol.* 1974;99:247–251.

3. Kirchner, JA. Glottic-supraglottic barrier: fact or fantasy? *Ann Otol Rhinol Laryngol.* 1997;106(8):700–704.

4. Laccourreye H, Laccourreye O, Weinstein G, Menard M, Brasnu D. Supracricoid laryngectomy with cricohyoidopexy: a partial laryngeal procedure for selected supraglottic and transglottic carcinomas. *Laryngoscope.* 1990;100:735–741.

5. Pearson BW. Near total laryngectomy. In: Silver CE, ed. *Atlas of Head and Neck Surgery.* New York: Churchill Livingstone; 1986:235–251

6. deVincentiis M, Minni A, Gallo A. Supracricoid laryngectomy with cricohyoidopexy (CHP) in the treatment of laryngeal cancer: a functional and oncologic experience. *Laryngoscope.* 1996;106:1108–1114.

7. Sato K, Kurita S, Hirano M. Location of the pre-epiglottic space and its relationship to the paraglottic space. *Ann Otol Rhinol Laryngol.* 1993;102:930–934.

SUPRAGLOTTIC CANCER

The ventricle marks the boundary between the glottic and supraglottic parts of the larynx. Each has its own blood supply and lymphatic drainage pattern, virtually independent of one another. The division makes it possible, in properly selected cases, to resect carcinoma in one of these divisions while sparing the other. Except for the ventricle, an anatomic barrier that would prevent the spread of carcinoma from the supraglottis to the glottis has never been identified. Nevertheless, most squamous cell carcinoma that arises on the supraglottic mucosa remains confined above the ventricle, resulting in the high rate of local control with horizontal supraglottic laryngectomy in properly selected cases.[1]

Cancer at the base of the epiglottis invades the preepiglottic space early in its development,[2] but it does not invade the thyroid cartilage. Of 112 supraglottic lesions in the Yale collection, the thyroid lamina was not invaded in a single specimen.[3] The intact thyroid cartilage allows saw cuts to be made safely during horizontal supraglottic laryngectomy. In those tumors originating supraglottically but extending to the floor of the ventricle, true cord or across the anterior commissure ("transglottic" in our practice) supracricoid laryngectomy may be useful, because it removes the thyroid cartilage which is likely to be invaded in such cases.[4]

Of 282 patients with supraglottic cancer treated between 1962 and 1989 at Yale-New Haven Hospital, 104 had clinically positive nodes on admission, and in 30 others, positive nodes are known to have appeared later (48% in all).[5]

Patterns of spread from the primary lesion are shown in the following sections.

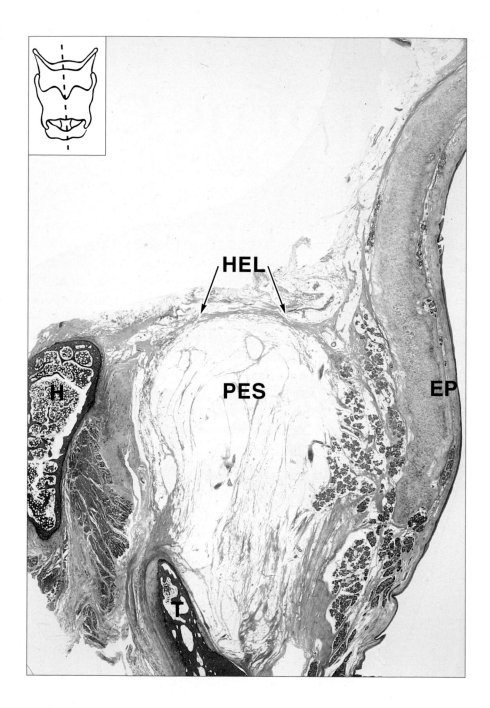

PLATE 69. Midsagittal section, normal supraglottic larynx. The hyoepiglottic ligament (HEL) forms the roof of the preepiglottic space (PES), filled mainly with fat. This space is usually invaded by cancer originating at the base of the epiglottis (EP). H = hyoid bone T = thyroid cartilage

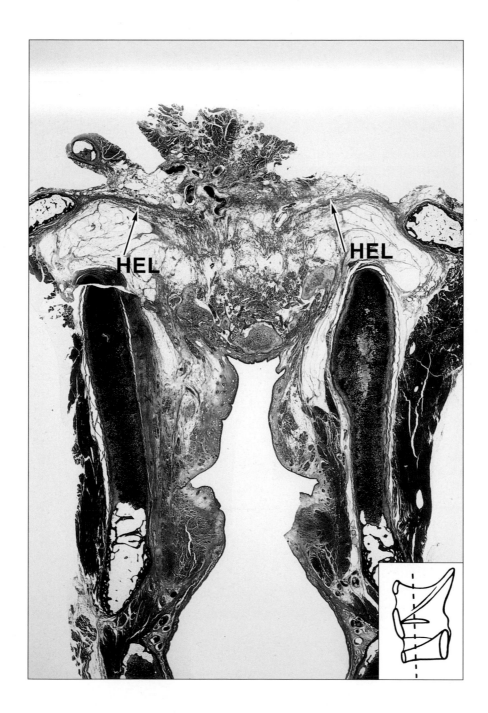

PLATE 70. Coronal section of a normal larynx, showing hyoepiglottic ligament (HEL) acting as the roof of the preepiglottic space. A small amount of muscle at the base of the tongue is seen above the ligament.

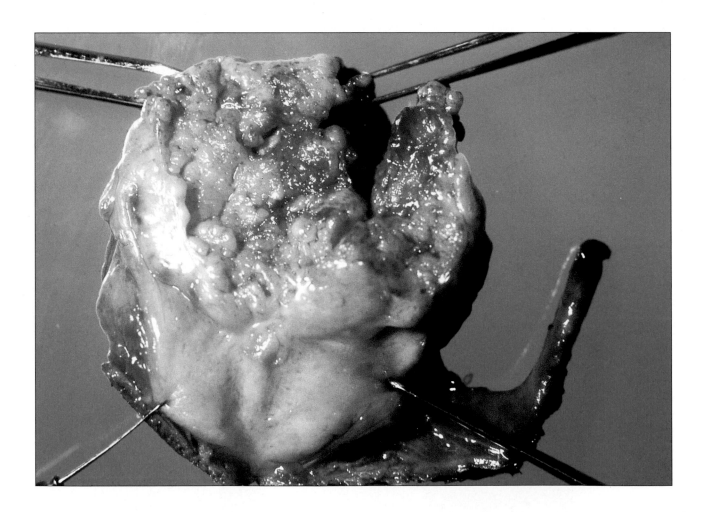

PLATE 71. Supraglottic laryngectomy specimen with carcinoma at the free edge of the epiglottis. The lower edge of the tumor is still above the level of the hyoid bone, a useful reference in clinical evaluation of epiglottic carcinoma. The level of the hyoid bone corresponds closely to that of the hyoepiglottic ligament, the real barrier to the spread of tumor into the base of the tongue during its early stages. (Reprinted from Kirchner, JA. Relationship of the Pathologist to the Laryngologist. In: A Ferlito *Surgical Pathology of Laryngeal Neoplasms* [Fig 1-2]. London. Chapman and Hall Medical, © 1996, with permission.)

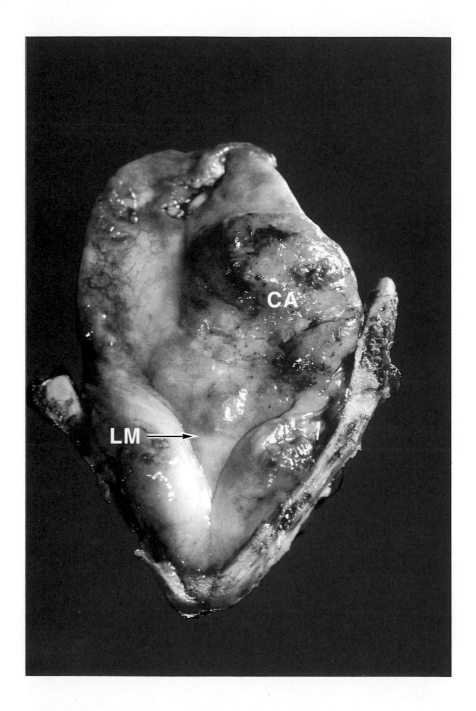

PLATE 72. Supraglottic laryngectomy specimen of tumor (CA) at midepiglottis and along the right ary- epiglottic fold. The lower edge (LM) of the tumor is shown, with an adequate margin immediately below.

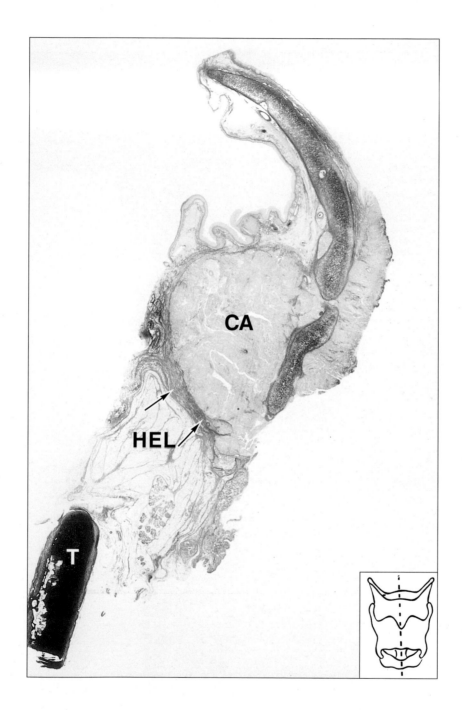

PLATE 73. Midsagittal section of the previous specimen. The tumor (CA) remains above the hyoepiglottic ligament (HEL), spreads submucosally into the vallecula and does not invade the preepiglottic space. T = thyroid cartilage. (Reprinted from Kirchner JA. Spread and Barriers to Spread of Cancer within the Larynx. In: Silver CE, ed. *Laryngeal Cancer* [Fig 2-7]. New York: Thieme, © 1991, with permission.)

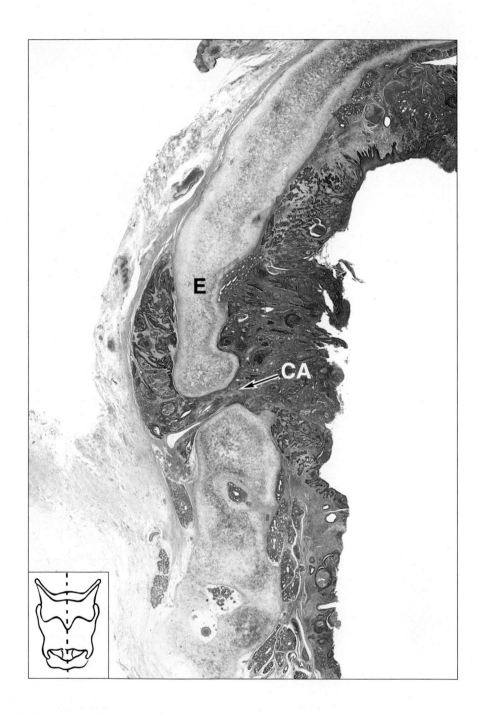

PLATE 74. Midsagittal section of a different specimen. Carcinoma (CA) on the laryngeal surface of the epiglottis (E) often spreads into the preepiglottic space through the fenestrae in the epiglottic cartilage (arrow).

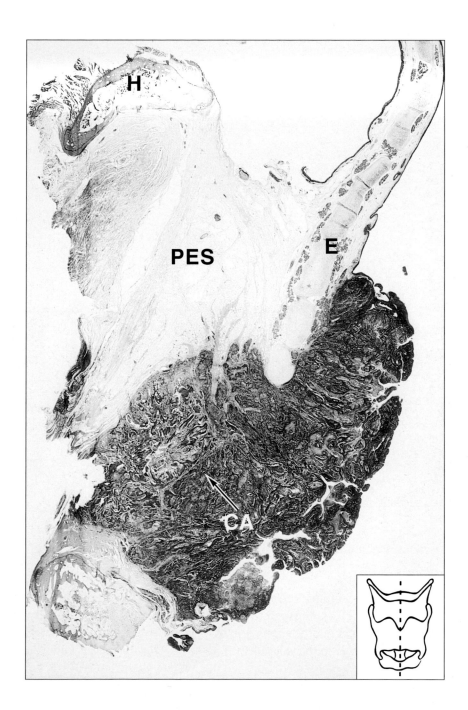

PLATE 75. Midsagittal section from a different specimen. Carcinoma (CA) may invade the preepiglottic space (PES) through the thyroepiglottic ligament, largely destroyed in this specimen. H = hyoid bone E = epiglottis

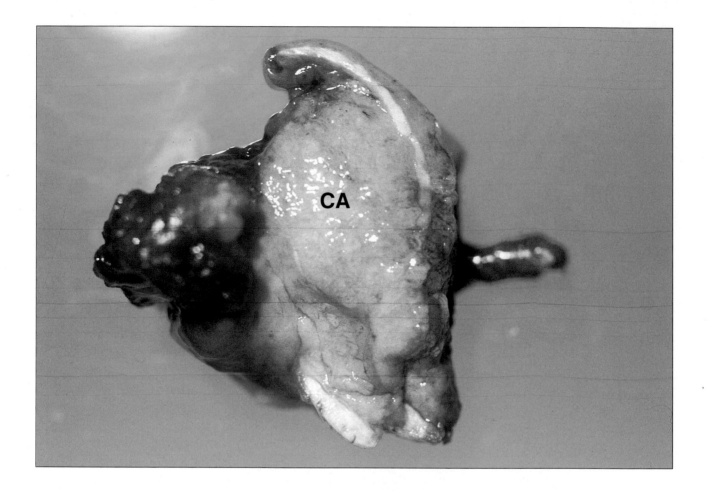

PLATE 76. Supraglottic laryngectomy specimen illustrating the spread of carcinoma (CA) through the thyroepiglottic ligament into the preepiglottic space. A smooth submucosal bulge was palpable in the vallecula. The tumor has not extended into the base of the tongue. The contents of the preepiglottic space can be removed as completely by supraglottic as by total laryngectomy. (Reprinted from Kirchner JA. Staging in Cancer of the Larynx. In: *Otolaryngology* Vol 5 [Ch 35, Fig 4]. Philadelphia: Lippincott-Raven, © 1979, with permission.)

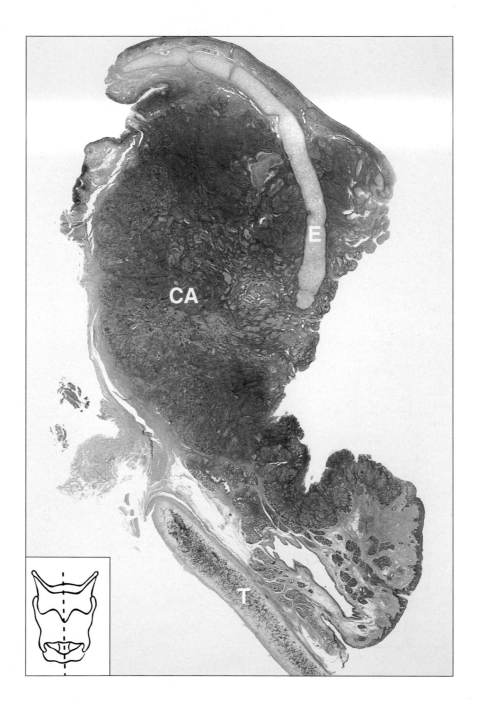

PLATE 77. Midsagittal section of the previous specimen. The hyoid bone was removed from the specimen before processing. The thyroepiglottic ligament below the epiglottic cartilage has been destroyed by the advancing cancer. The base of the tongue was uninvolved. Radical neck dissection produced 19 lymph nodes, 2 of which contained metastatic carcinoma. The patient survived, free of disease, for more than 15 years. T = thyroid cartilage E = epiglottis CA = cancer (Reprinted from Kirchner JA. Horizontal Partial Resections of the Larynx—Posttherapeutic Histology and Microstaging. In: Wigand ME, Steiner W, Stell PM, eds. *Functional Partial Laryngectomy* [Fig 3, p 210]. New York: Springer-Verlag, © 1984, with permission.)

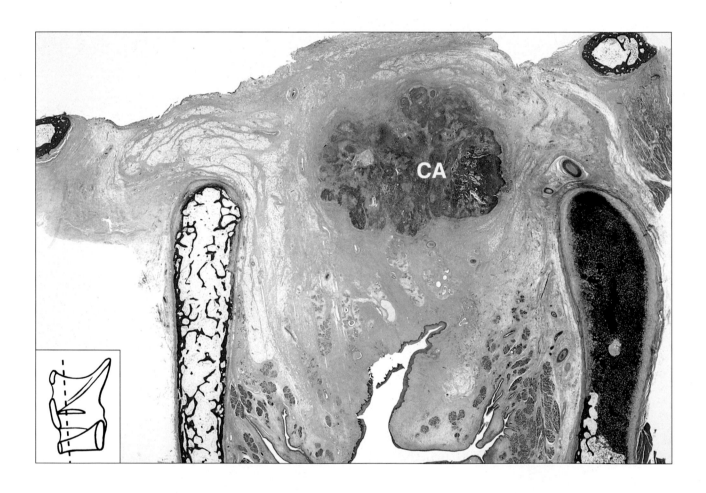

PLATE 78. Coronal section of a different specimen treated unsuccessfully by full-course irradiation for cancer at the base of the epiglottis. Residual carcinoma (CA) and necrotic tumor are the usual findings in preepiglottic space tumor treated by irradiation. The upper part of the right thyroid ala remains unossified in this specimen. The patient, a 56-year-old white male, showed no evidence of disease 10 years after total laryngectomy.

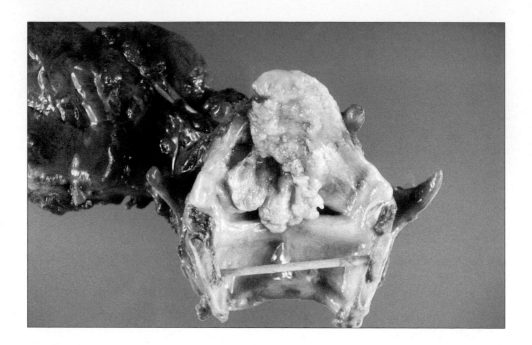

PLATE 79. A supraglottic tumor may present a "shaggy" surface as shown here and conceal enough of the true cords to suggest transglottic spread. Of importance, however, is the absence of tumor behind the ventricle at the arytenoid area. This area is almost always involved in transglottic cancer.

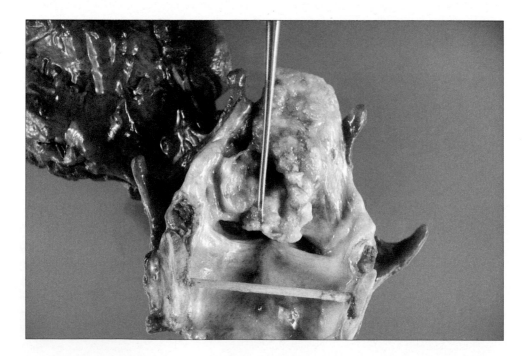

PLATE 80. The true cords are free of visible tumor. Apart from local anatomic contraindications to supraglottic laryngectomy, the patient's medical condition, especially the pulmonary reserve, may dictate a total, rather than partial, laryngectomy. (Reprinted from Kirchner JA. Treatment of Laryngeal Cancer. In: Chretien PB et al, eds. *Head and Neck Cancer* Vol. 1 [Fig 2, p 200]. Philadelphia/Toronto: BC Decker, Inc., © 1985, with permission.)

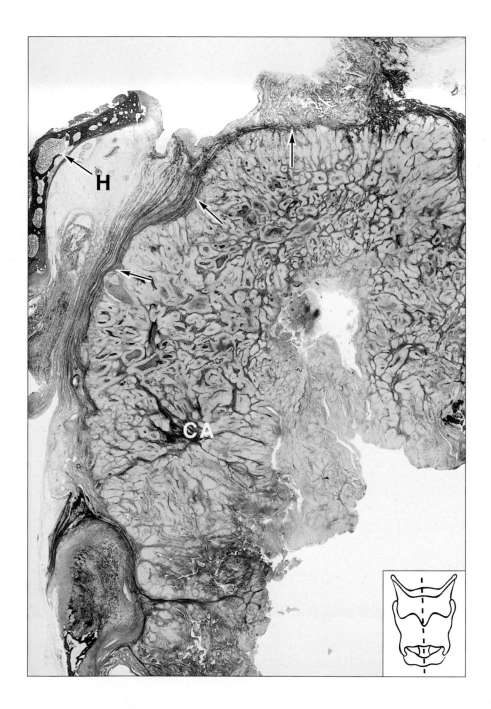

PLATE 81. Midsagittal section of the previous specimen stained for elastic tissue. Cancer invading the preepiglottic space is usually confined by a fibro-elastic membrane (arrows), resulting in a tumor-free area between the hyoid bone (H) and the advancing edge of tumor. The tumor-free space allows preservation of the hyoid bone, a more secure closure of the pharyngotomy, and earlier rehabilitation of deglutition. The tumor-free space also facilitates cricohyoidopexy in cases where such surgery is indicated.[4] CA = cancer

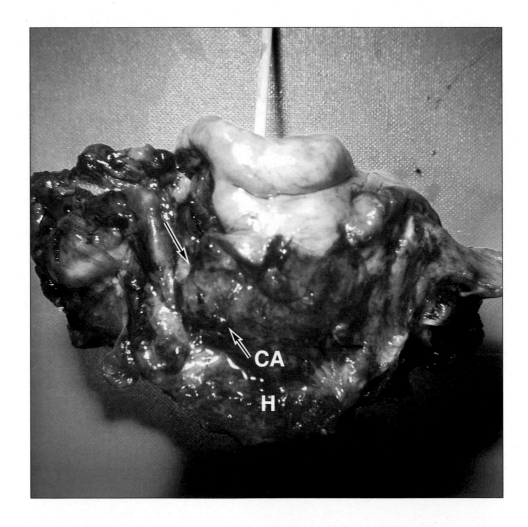

PLATE 82. Total laryngectomy specimen viewed from above. A smooth, indurated area was palpable in the vallecula (CA). H = hyoid bone°

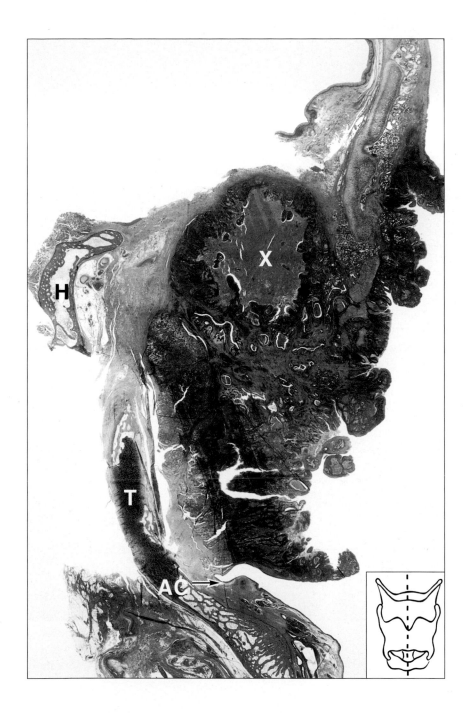

PLATE 83. Midsagittal section of the previous specimen. The tumor approaches the base of the tongue but has not breached the hyoepiglottic ligament. The usual tumor-free space is seen between the hyoid bone (H) and the advancing edge of the tumor. Necrosis (X) just below the hyoepiglottic ligament is typical of many large tumors in the pre-epiglottic fat pad, possibly related to its sparse blood supply. T = thyroid cartilage AC = anterior commissure (Reprinted from Mancuso AA, Hanafee WN, [Contributor: JA Kirchner]. Laryngeal Trauma and Other Benign Lesions. *Computed Tomography of the Head & Neck*, 2nd ed [Ch 9, Fig 9.32). Baltimore: Williams & Wilkins, © 1985, with permission.)

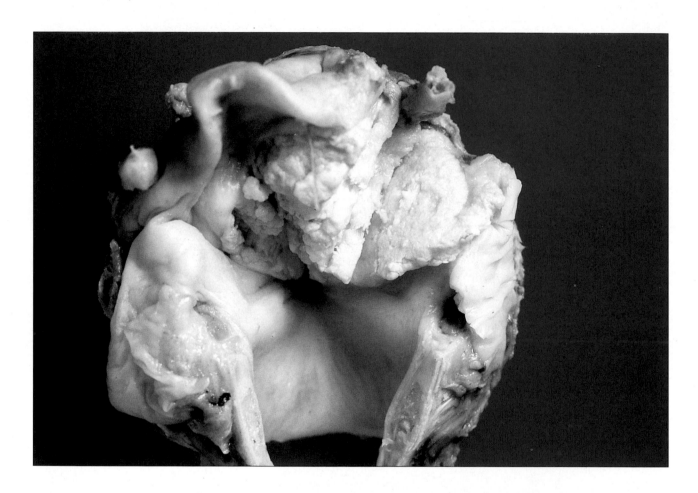

PLATE 84. A large supraglottic carcinoma removed by total laryngectomy with induration palpable in the thyrohyoid membrane.

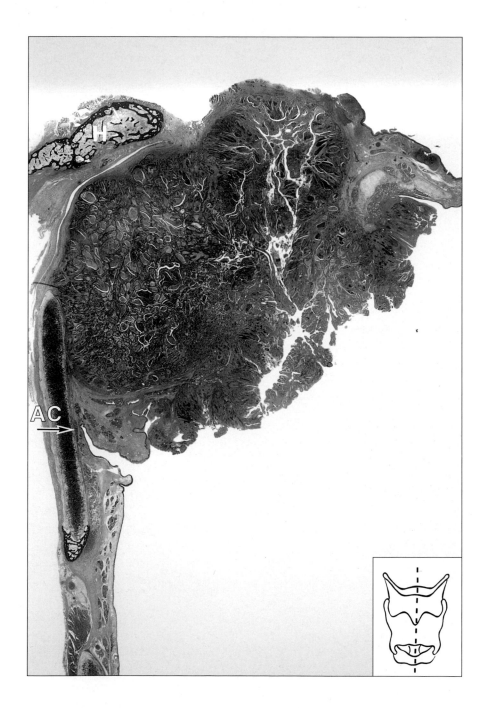

PLATE 85. Midsagittal section of the previous specimen showing carcinoma in the preepiglottic space, abutting the hyoid bone (H). At total laryngectomy, the palpable mass behind the thyrohyoid membrane and in the base of the tongue required removal of the hyoid (H) with the specimen. Resection of the hyoid bone was mandatory in only 4 of 71 supraglottic specimens suitably sectioned to show this relationship. AC = anterior commissure

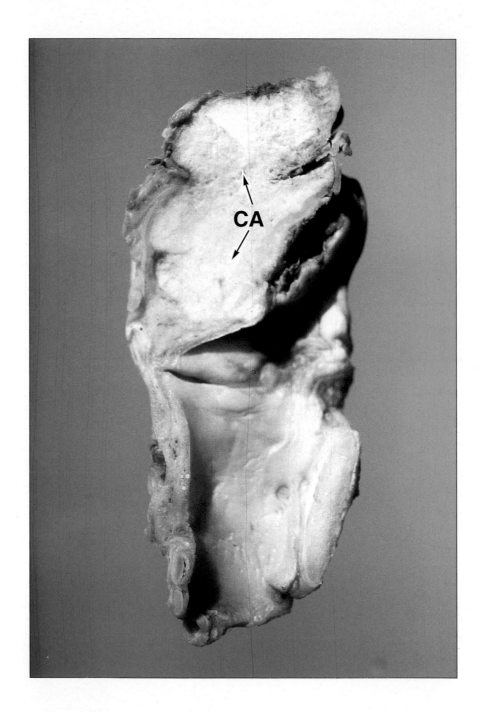

PLATE 86. Supraglottic carcinoma (CA) invading the base of the tongue. The specimen had been fixed in formalin.

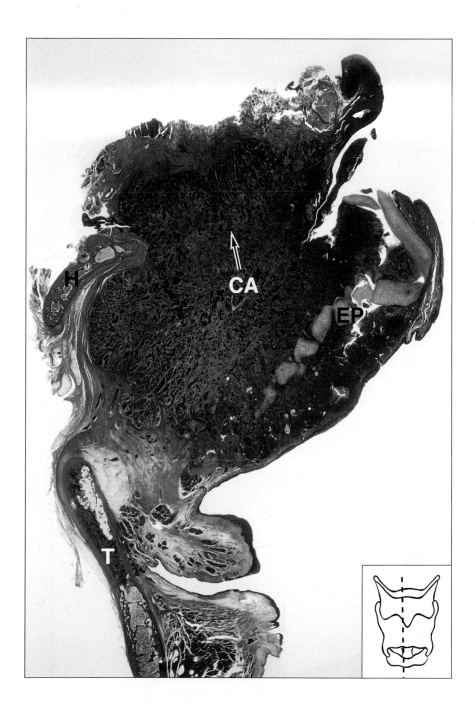

PLATE 87. Parasagittal section of the previous specimen. The hyoepiglottic ligament has been breached and tongue musculature invaded. In this and three other specimens, proximity of tumor to the hyoid bone (H) required its removal, although the bone itself was not invaded. Palpable induration in the vallecula or thyrohyoid membrane requires removal of the hyoid bone as part of the specimen. T = thyroid cartilage CA = cancer EP = base of epiglottis

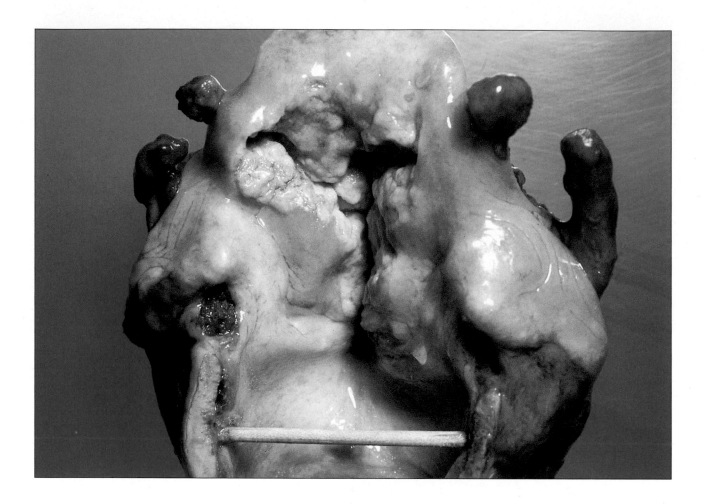

PLATE 88. Carcinoma involving most of the supraglottic larynx. The true cord was not visible before the operation.

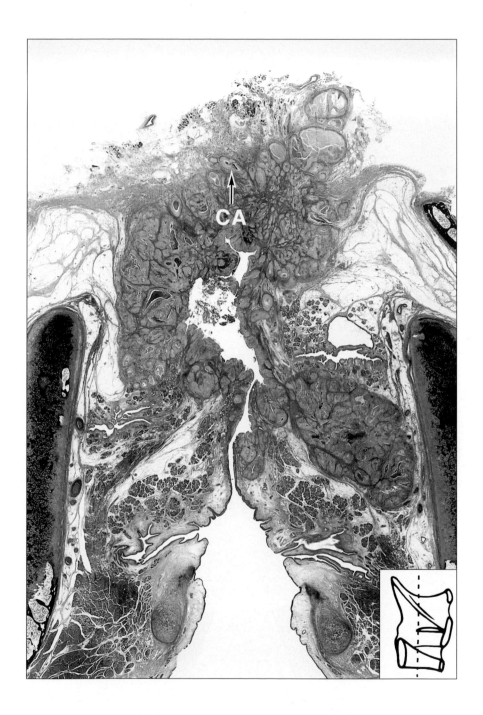

PLATE 89. Coronal section of the previous specimen. Elastic tissue stain shows carcinoma (CA) invading the base of the tongue and destruction of the hyo-epiglottic ligament at this plane.

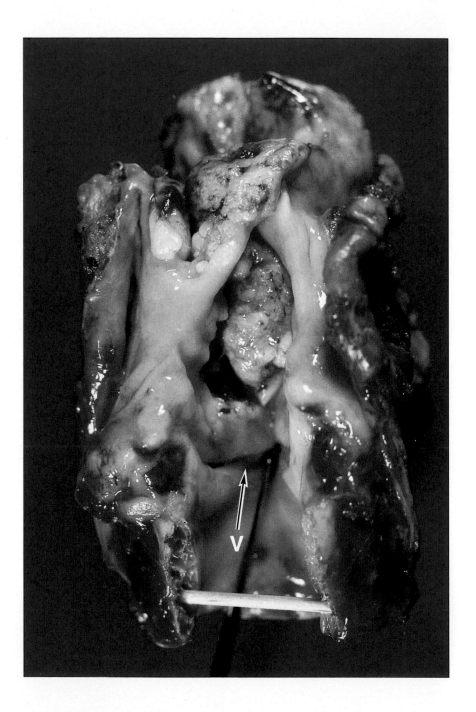

PLATE 90. Bilateral supraglottic carcinoma. The ventricle (V) remains free of tumor. The specimen was divided in the midline, the right side sectioned sagitally, the left side coronally.

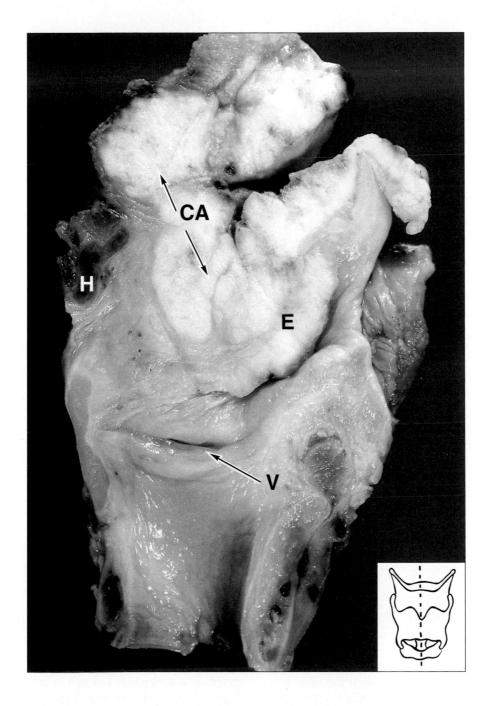

PLATE 91. Right half showing the tumor (CA) extending from the epiglottis (E) into the preepiglottic space and base of the tongue. The ventricle (V) is free of tumor. H = hyoid bone

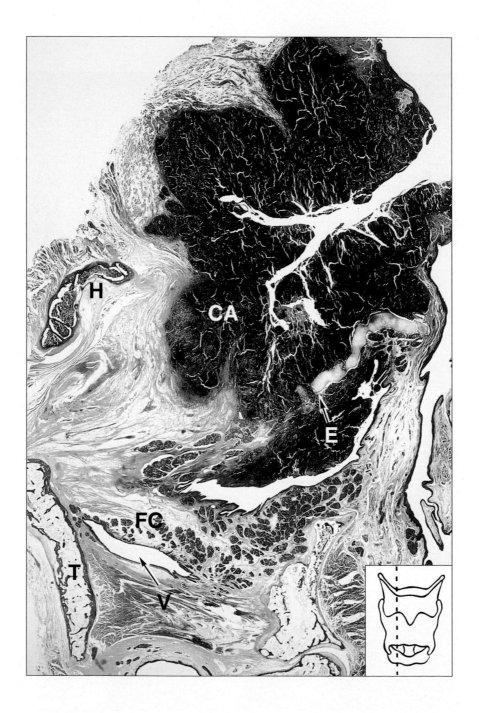

PLATE 92. Parasagittal section of the right half of the specimen. The cancer (CA) spreads from the laryngeal surface of the epiglottis (E) into the preepiglottic space. The ventricle (V), is free of tumor. FC = false cord H = hyoid bone T = thyroid cartilage

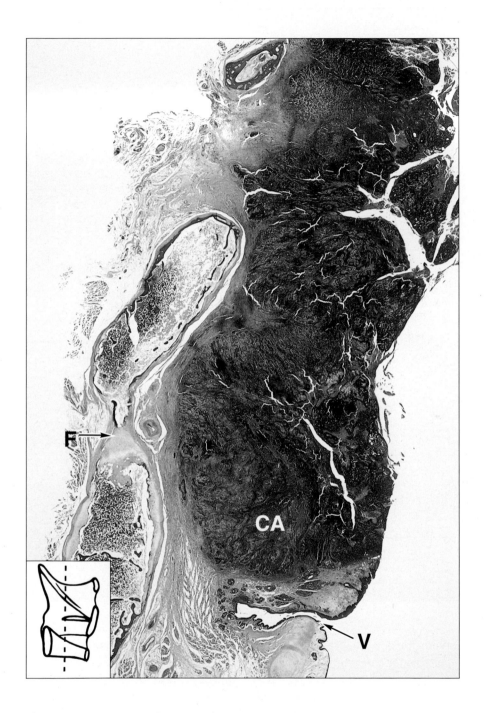

PLATE 93. Coronal section, left half of the previous specimen. Ventricle (V) and the true cord are free of cancer (CA). A normal fenestra (F) in the thyroid cartilage is seen at the arrow. The adjacent blood vessel passes through the fenestra in other planes. The fenestra was found in 39% of coronally sectioned specimens in the collection (47/121). Unlike invasion through the epiglottic foramina, adjacent cancer was not found to traverse the fenestra in a single specimen.[6] (Reprinted from Kirchner JA. Spread and Barriers to Spread of Cancer within the Larynx. In: Silver CE, ed. *Laryngeal Cancer* [Fig 2-9]. New York: Thieme, © 1991, with permission.)

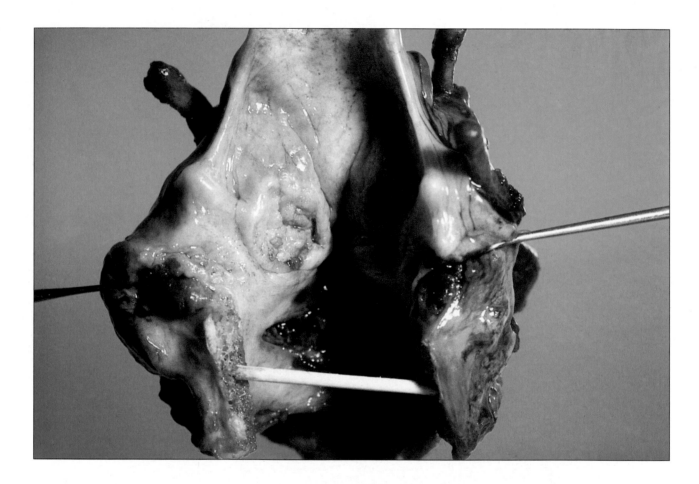

PLATE 94. False cord lesion. Its proximity to the arytenoid made it unsuitable for conventional supraglottic laryngectomy. Removal of an arytenoid as a means of obtaining an adequate margin is oncologically sound, but removing it because of overlying carcinoma, fixation, or induration may cut across tumor spreading submucosally into the true cord.

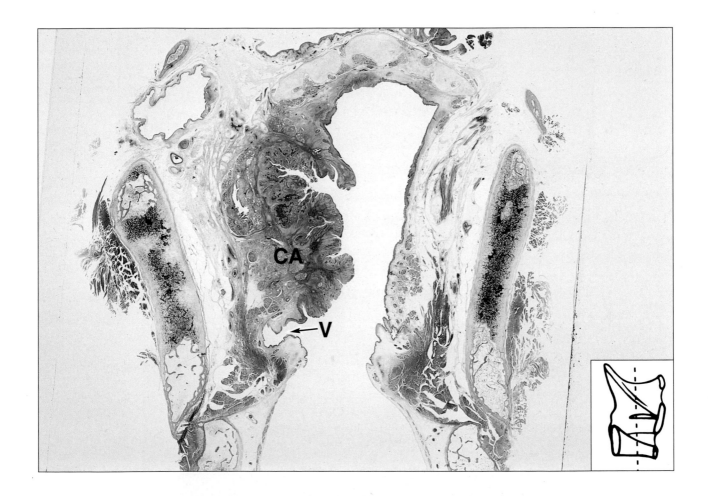

PLATE 95. Coronal section of the previous specimen. The ventricle (V) and true cord are free of tumor. Thyroid cartilage remains intact, a characteristic feature of supraglottic cancer. CA = cancer

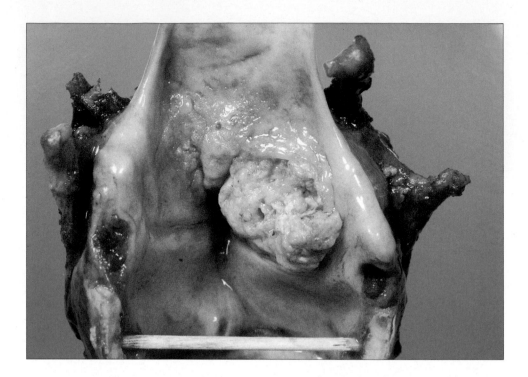

PLATE 96. Supraglottic carcinoma removed by total laryngectomy. Its bulk concealed the true cord on direct laryngoscopy, with the result that the lesion was classed as transglottic before the operation.

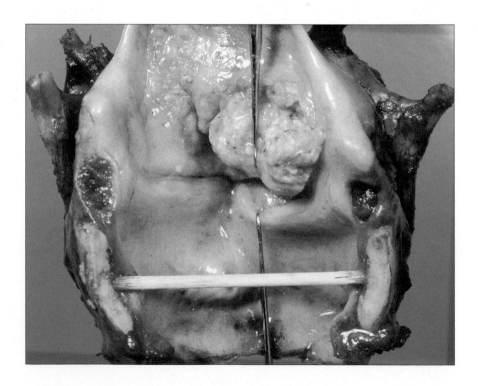

PLATE 97. The tumor is supraglottic, with the true cords and ventricles free of tumor on inspection. (Reprinted from Kirchner JA. The Systems of UICC and AJC for Staging of Laryngeal Carcinoma. In: Wigand ME, Steiner W, Stell PM, eds. *Functional Partial Laryngectomy* [Fig 4, p 72]. New York: Springer-Verlag, ©1984, with permission.)

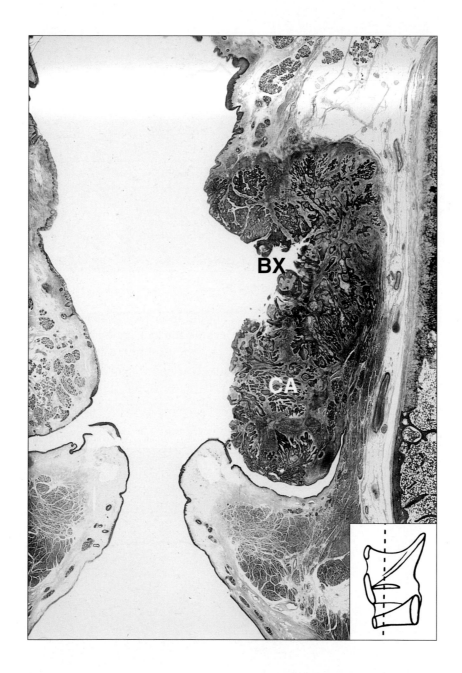

PLATE 98. Coronal sections show the true cord to be free of tumor at this and other planes. Biopsy site is seen at BX. The lesion could possibly have been resected by horizontal supraglottic laryngectomy, but this 72-year-old patient's pulmonary reserve was marginal. CA = cancer (Reprinted from Kirchner JA. The Systems of UICC and AJC for Staging of Laryngeal Carcinoma. In: Wigand ME, Steiner W, Stell PM, eds. *Functional Partial Laryngectomy* [Fig 5, p 73]. New York: Springer-Verlag, ©1984, with permission.)

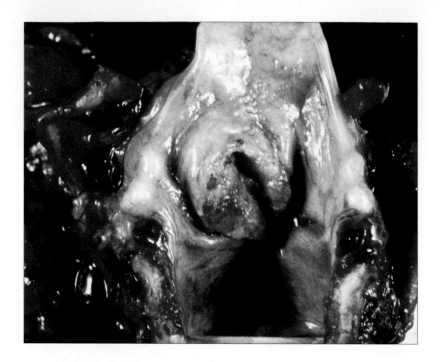

PLATE 99. Supraglottic carcinoma arising in the angle between the false cord and base of epiglottis. Termed "Winkelkarzinom" in German literature, the "angle carcinoma" is characterized by the deep cleft seen in this tumor.[7] Because of its bulk, such lesions often overhang and conceal the true cord. The cleft, however, should indicate the supraglottic nature of the tumor, even if the true cord cannot be seen on indirect laryngoscopy. (Reprinted from Ariyan S. *Cancer of the Head and Neck* [Fig 15-5]. St. Louis: CV Mosby Inc., © 1987, with permission.)

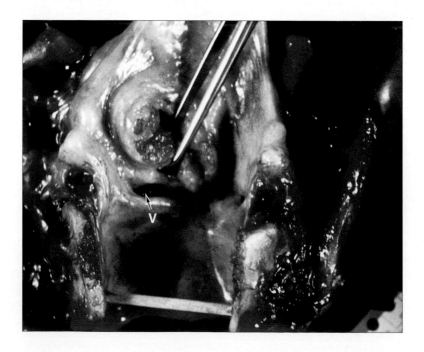

PLATE 100. The lower edge of the tumor does not invade the ventricle (V). The true cord is uninvolved, the arytenoid area free of visible tumor, and the lesion probably resectable by supraglottic laryngectomy. (Reprinted from Ariyan S. *Cancer of the Head and Neck* [Fig 15-6]. St. Louis: CV Mosby Inc., © 1987, with permission.)

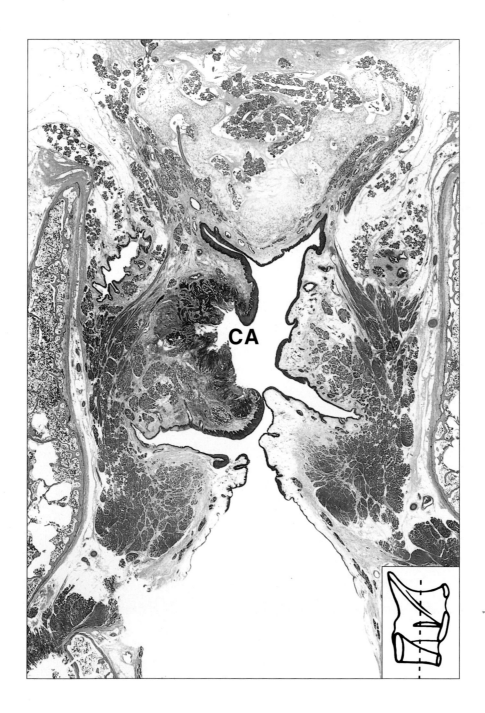

PLATE 101.   Coronal section of the previous specimen. The ventricle and true cord are free of tumor. CA = cancer

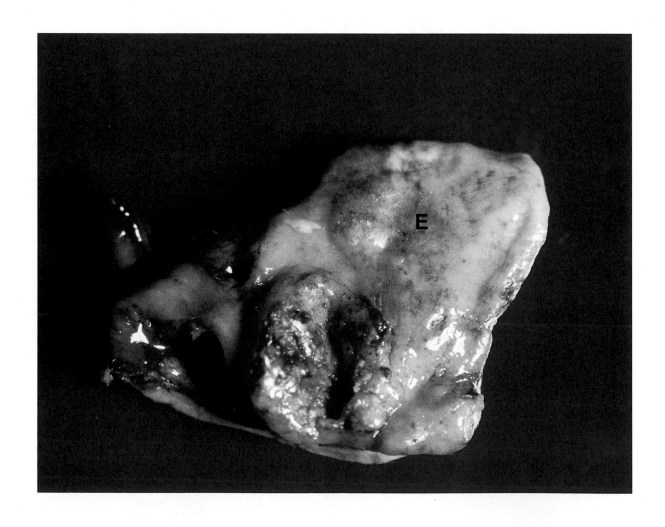

PLATE 102. Subtotal supraglottic laryngectomy specimen showing angle tumor with the characteristic vertical cleft. The epiglottis has been split near the midline, the arytenoid cartilage removed in order to obtain an adequate margin around the tumor, and the true cord sutured to the cricoid plate in the midline. Postoperative irradiation was followed by hypothyroidism. There was no recurrence of carcinoma after a 3-year follow-up. The pushing edge of most tumors in the preepiglottic space allows safe resection of that portion of the preepiglottic fat containing palpable tumor. E = epiglottis

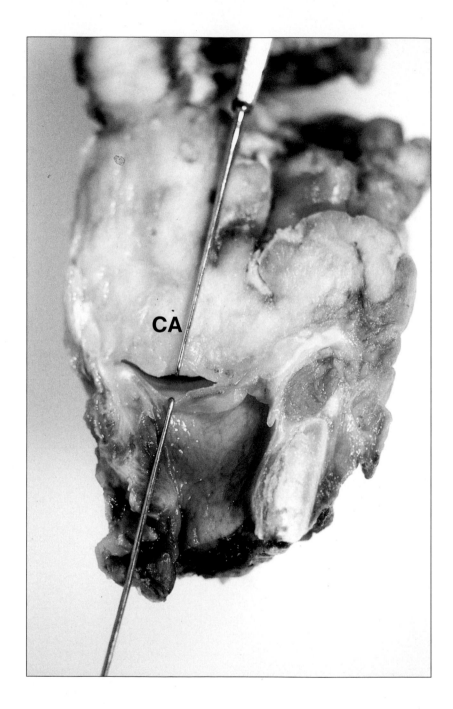

PLATE 103. This laryngectomy specimen was acquired after whole-organ sectioning was no longer available. Cancer (CA) had invaded the base of the tongue and extended into the hypopharynx. Multiple sections through the thyroid cartilage were prepared by the pathologist, with none of the sections showing invasion. This specimen is included as an extreme example of the principle that carcinoma limited to the supraglottis does not invade the thyroid cartilage.[3]

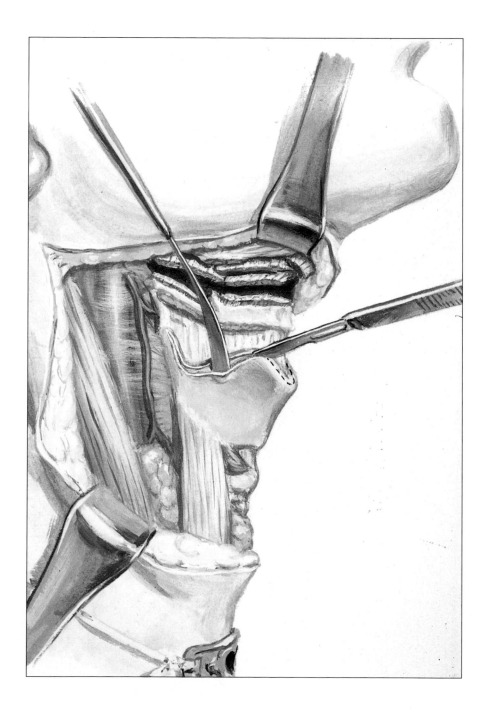

PLATE 104. In those supraglottic carcinomas suitable for supraglottic laryngectomy, the tumor-free thyroid cartilage allows safe elevation of the external perichondrium. (This illustration and the ones in Plates 105 and 106 were prepared by the late Frank Netter for inclusion in Reference 8.)

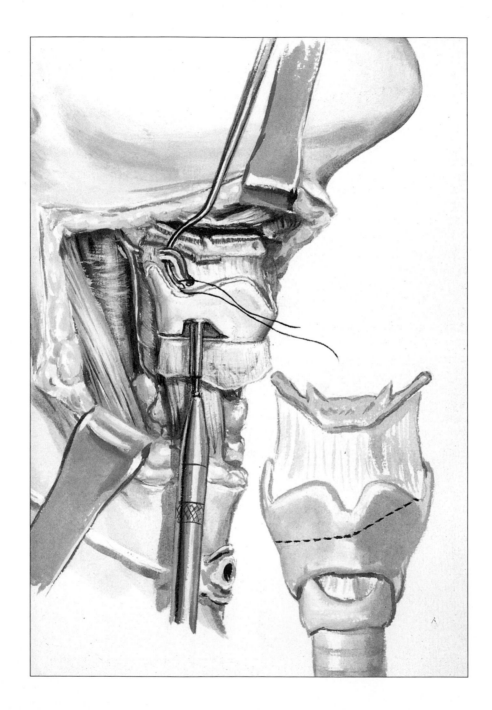

PLATE 105. The intact thyroid ala allows the saw cut to be made safely at the level of the ventricle.

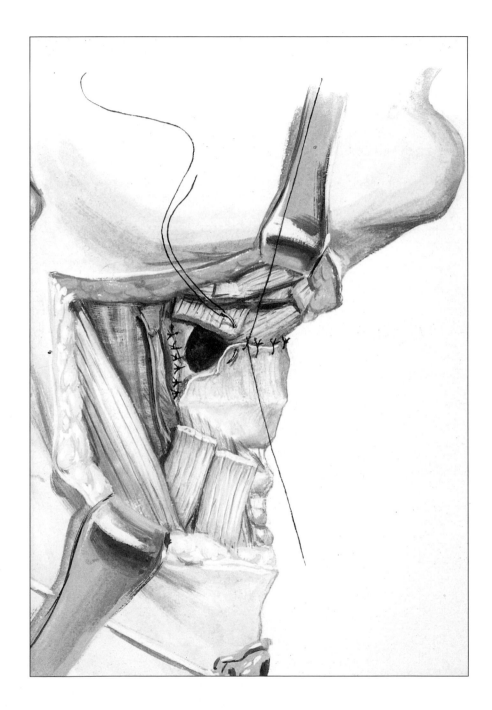

PLATE 106. Because the cartilage itself is free of tumor, the external perichondrium can be safely used for repair of the pharyngotomy.

REFERENCES

1. Kirchner JA. Glottic-supraglottic barrier: fact or fantasy? *Ann Otol Rhinol Laryngol.* 1997;106(8):700–704.
2. Zeitels SM, Vaughan CW. Preepiglottic space invasion in "early" epiglottic cancer. *Ann Otol Rhinol Laryngol.* 1991;100:789–792.
3. Kirchner JA. What have whole organ sections contributed to the treatment of laryngeal cancer? *Ann Otol Rhinol Laryngol.* 1989;98:661–667.
4. Laccourreye O, Brasnu D, Merite-Drancy A, Cauchois R, Chabardes E, Menard M, Laccourreye H. Cricohyoidopexy in selected infrahyoid epiglottic carcinomas presenting with pathological preepiglottic space invasion. *Arch Otolaryngol Head & Neck Surgery.* 1993; 119(8):881–6.
5. Kirchner JA. Controversies in the management of T3 supraglottic cancer. In: Fee WE, Goepfert H, Johns ME, Strong EW, Ward PH, eds. *Head and Neck Cancer,* Philadelphia, Toronto: B.C. Decker, Inc; 1990;130–133.
6. Kirchner JC, Kirchner JA, Sasaki CT. Anatomic foramina in the thyroid cartilage: incidence and implications for the spread of laryngeal cancer. *Ann Otol Rhinol Laryngol.* 1989;98:421–425.
7. Kleinsasser O. *Tumors of the Larynx and Hypopharynx,* New York: Thieme Medical Publishers, Inc; 1988:102.
8. Som M. Conservation surgery for carcinoma of the supraglottis. *J Laryng.* 1970;84:655–678.

HYPOPHARYNGEAL CANCER

The hypopharyngeal cancers included in this section are limited to those that invade the larynx or affect its function, viz. cancer of the pyriform sinus and postcricoid area.

Pyriform sinus cancer limited to the medial or upper lateral walls may be suitable for partial laryngectomy.[1] Such lesions have not invaded the framework in our specimens.[2] A small lesion of the lateral wall can be resected along with that portion of the thyroid ala that overlies the pyriform sinus. Medial wall tumors may be resected by a modification of the horizontal supraglottic technique after exposure by lateral pharyngotomy.[3]

A tumor infiltrating the anterior wall or "angle" of the pyriform sinus may invade the paraglottic and adjoining preepiglottic space. Because the anterior wall of the pyriform sinus abuts the paraglottic space,[4] invasion of this space allows the tumor to spread into both the supraglottic and the glottic larynx, while sparing the overlying laryngeal mucosa. The result may be swelling and induration of the false cord, sometimes the only visible evidence of tumor, because the pyriform sinus lesion may be small and the anterior wall difficult to visualize.

In advanced stages, pyriform sinus cancer invades the thyroid and cricoid cartilages, starting along the posterior edge of the thyroid cartilage, then infiltrating the cricoid. Invasion of the cricoid has been observed only in those pyriform sinus tumors that have invaded the apex.[2]

Limitation of motion or even complete immobility of the vocal cord without invasion of the endolarynx has been found in several pyriform sinus tumors and, in each case, was due to invasion of the posterior cricoarytenoid muscle.[5]

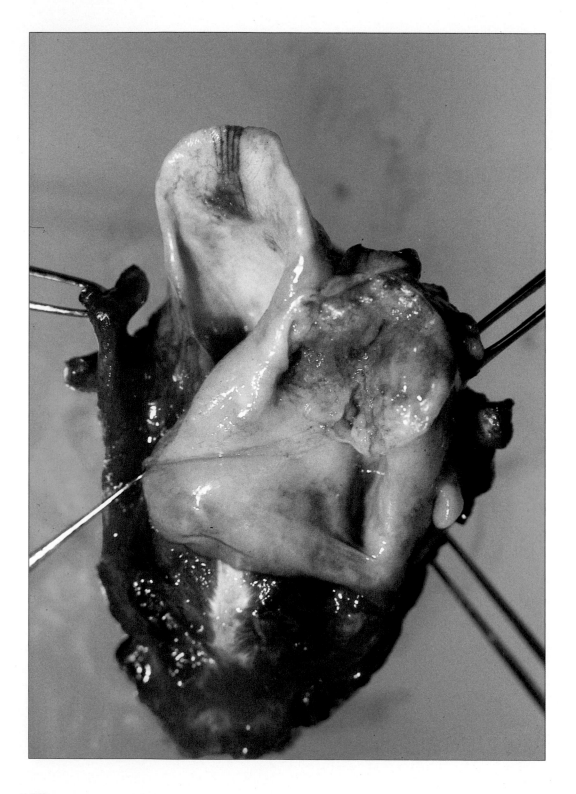

PLATE 107. Cancer in the upper right pyriform sinus. The apex is clear. Vocal cord mobility was normal.

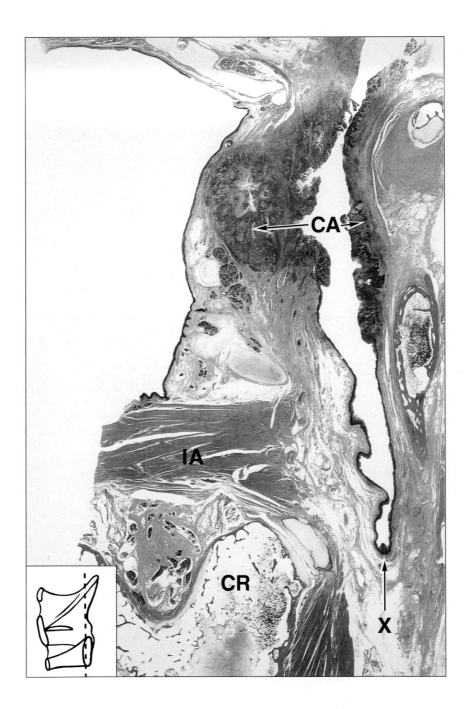

PLATE 108. Coronal section of the previous specimen. The tumor-free apex (vertical arrow at "X") indicates a very small likelihood of framework invasion.[2] Selected lesions of this type may be suitable for partial laryngectomy.[1,3] IA = interarytenoid muscle CR = cricoid plate CA = cancer

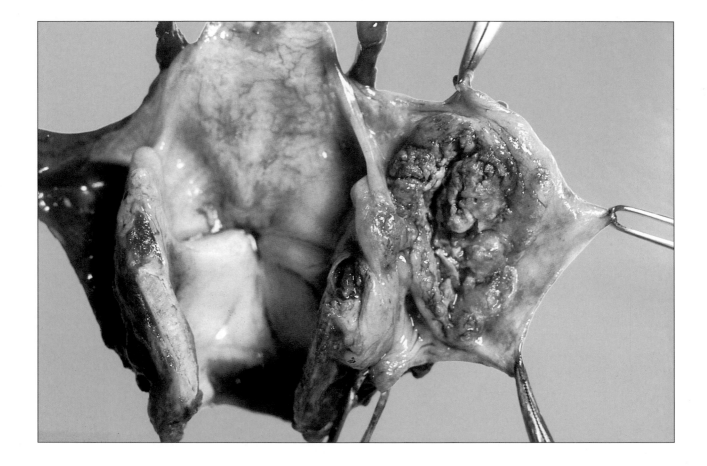

PLATE 109. Right pyriform sinus cancer similar to the previous lesion, but larger. It involves the medial wall, lateral wall, and the angle at which they meet. Pyriform sinus carcinoma in the anterior angle usually spreads submucosally into the soft tissues of the supra-glottic larynx. This specimen is exophytic and not likely to invade as deeply as an ulcerated tumor. (Reprinted from Kirchner JA, Carter D. The Larynx. In: Sternberg SS, ed. *Diagnostic Surgical Pathology* 2nd ed [Fig 27]. New York: Raven Press, © 1994, with permission.)

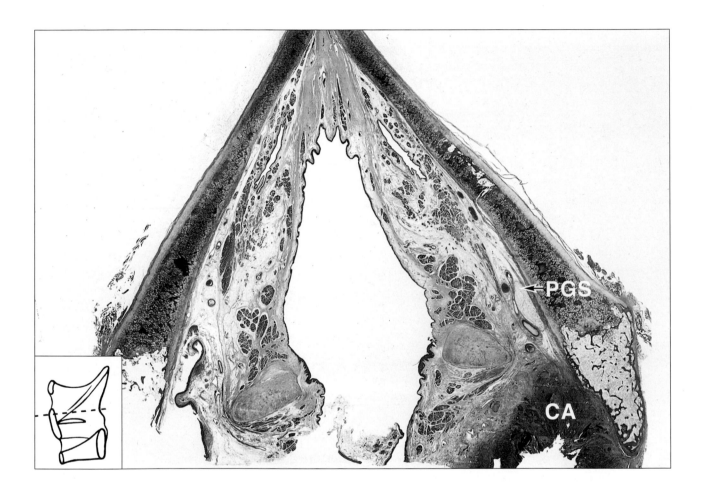

PLATE 110. Transverse section of the previous specimen. Cancer (CA) invades the supraglottic larynx along the inner surface of the thyroid cartilage, but has not extended into the paraglottic space (PGS), nor has it invaded the thyroid lamina.

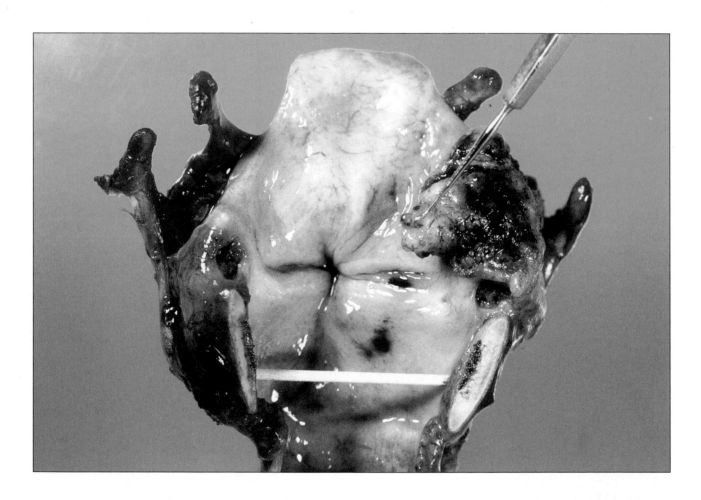

PLATE 111. Right pyriform sinus cancer extending over the aryepiglottic fold. The apex is not visible.

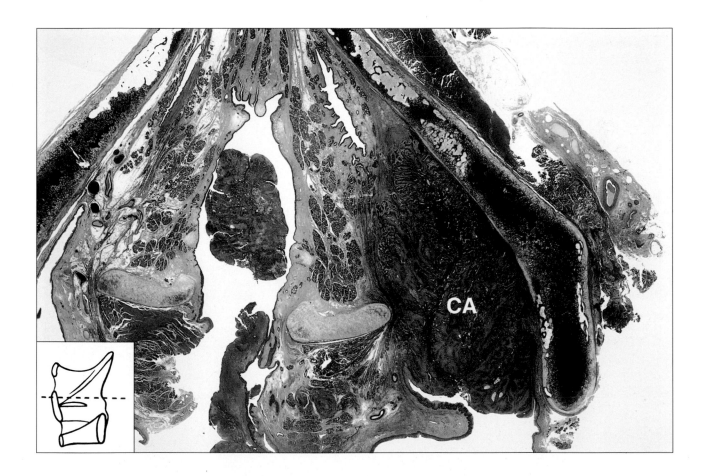

PLATE 112. In this horizontal section of the previous specimen, the lesion (CA) has spread into the supraglottic larynx but has not invaded the thyroid cartilage. Lack of ossification in this part of the specimen may be responsible. Cancer has filled the paraglottic space along the inner surface of the thyroid lamina.

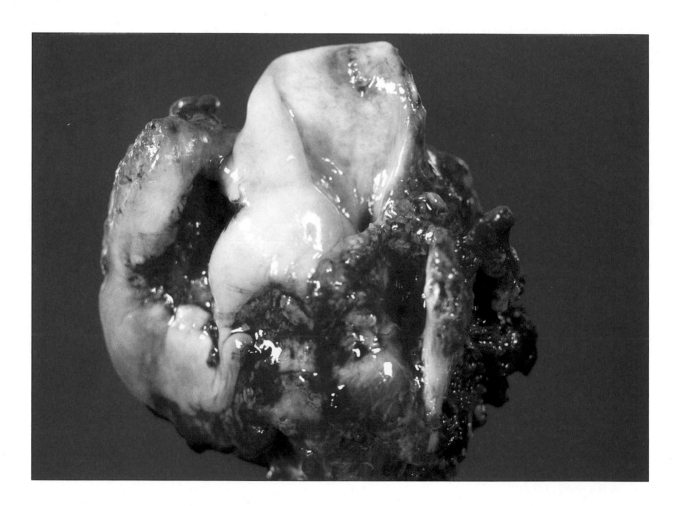

PLATE 113. Cancer in the right pyriform sinus, with deep invasion at the anterior angle.

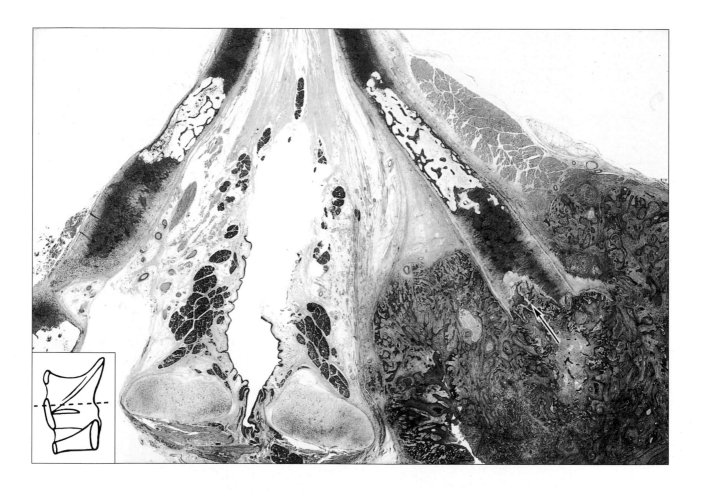

PLATE 114. Transverse section of the previous specimen showing invasion of the posterior edge of the thyroid cartilage (arrow). This feature indicates an unfavorable prognosis.[6]

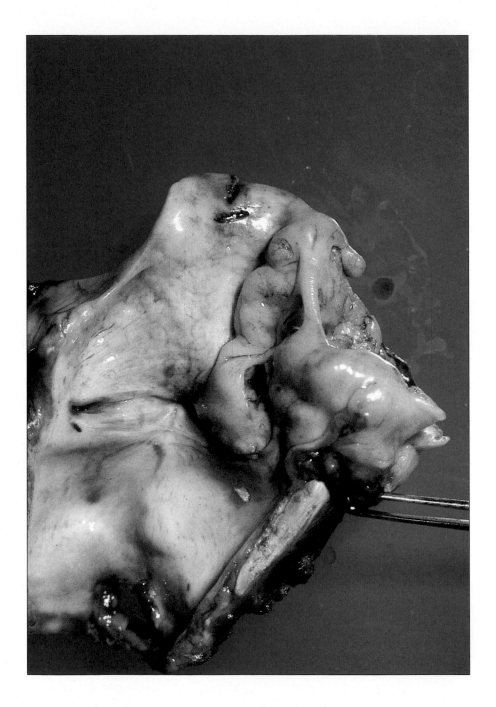

PLATE 115. Carcinoma of the right pyriform sinus with submucosal spread into the right aryepiglottic fold and false cord. Submucosal induration was palpable in the false cord and arytenoid area, with tumor visible in the pyriform sinus only after exposure by direct laryngoscopy. Induration at the arytenoid usually signals invasion of the glottic musculature from behind the ventricle.

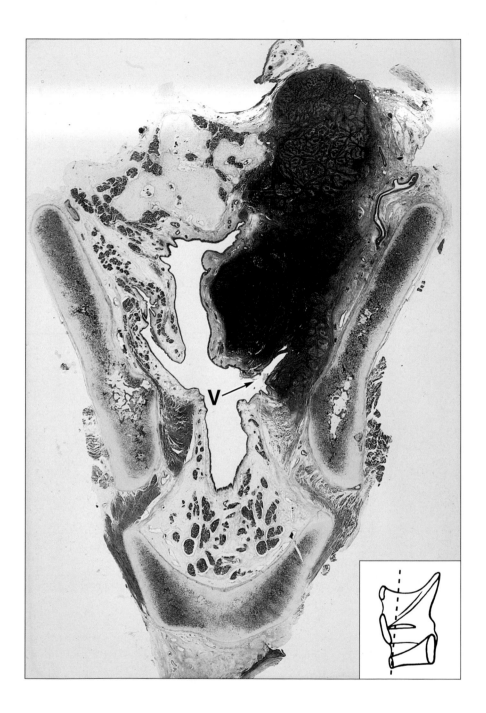

PLATE 116. Coronal section of the previous specimen at the anterior larynx. The tumor has invaded the supraglottic larynx, and has begun to spread into the glottic musculature by way of the paraglottic space, whose posterior edge contacts the pyriform sinus mucosa. Because the laryngeal portion of the tumor remains submucosal, the pyriform sinus proved to be the site of origin. The remaining ventricle (V) is being encircled from behind.

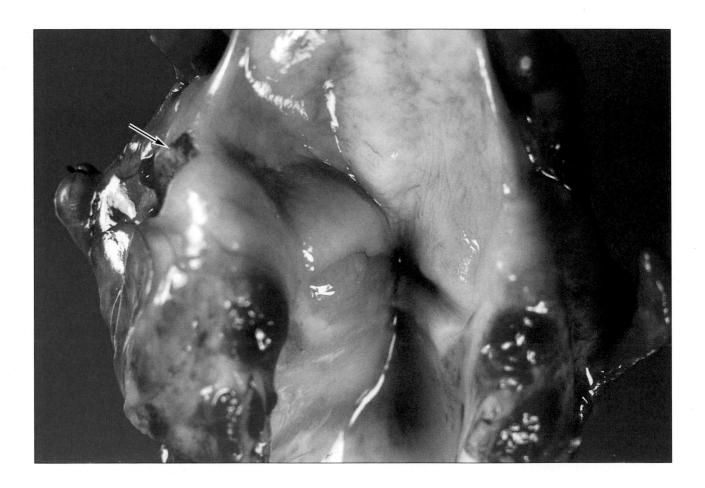

PLATE 117. This surgical specimen shows a tiny area of tumor at the arrow. Indirect laryngoscopy revealed massive edema of the arytenoid, ventricular band, and true cord, with no identifiable cancer. The patient's chief complaint was left-sided throat and ear pain.

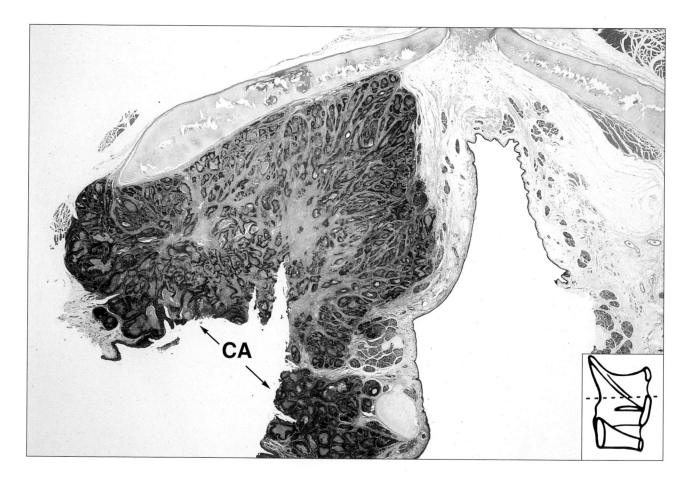

PLATE 118. Transverse section of the previous specimen. Most of this hypopharyngeal tumor is intralaryngeal, under intact mucosa. The tumor surface (arrows) was exposed when the surgical specimen was opened for closer inspection.

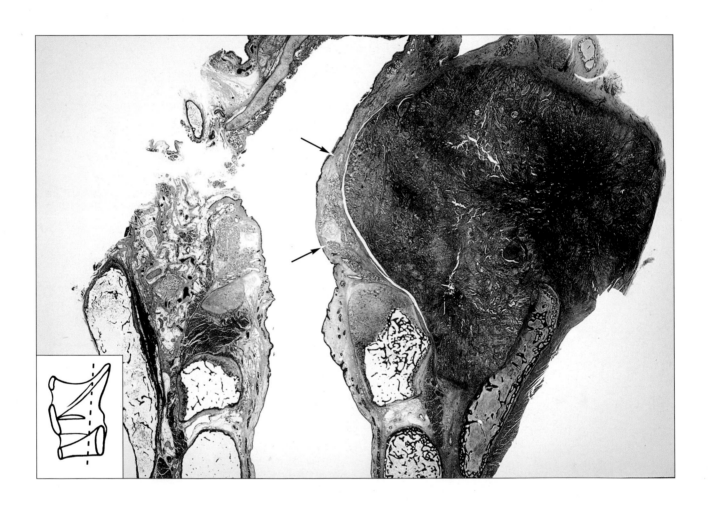

PLATE 119. Coronal section of a pyriform sinus carcinoma exhibiting a "pushing" edge. The tumor has displaced the overlying supraglottic mucosa (arrows). None of the lymph nodes in the radical neck dissection showed metastatic carcinoma. Compared to carcinoma with an infiltrating edge, carcinoma with a pushing edge produces fewer regional metastases.[7,8]

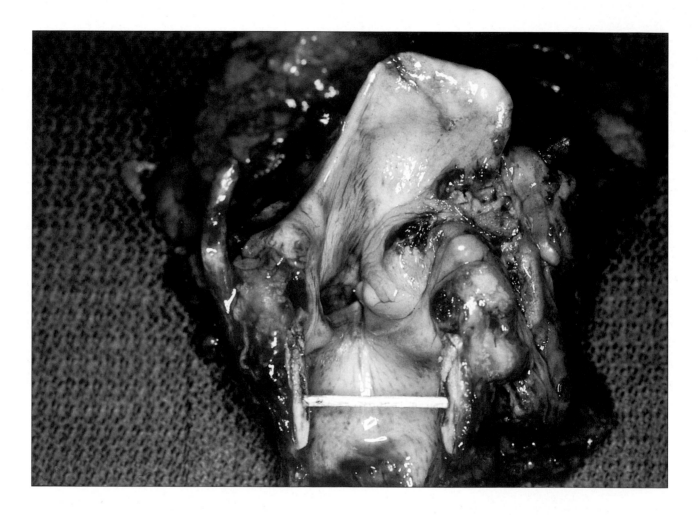

PLATE 120. Right pyriform sinus carcinoma extending over the aryepiglottic fold. The initial finding was a firm 2 × 2-cm mass in the neck, which moved when the patient swallowed. Obstructed airway required tracheotomy.

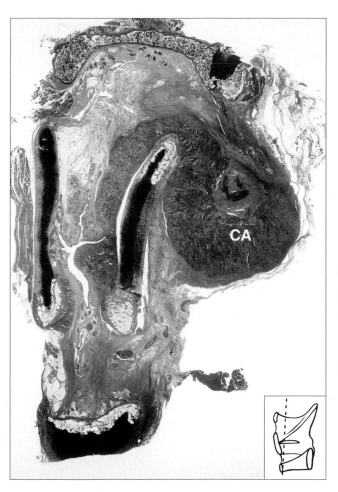

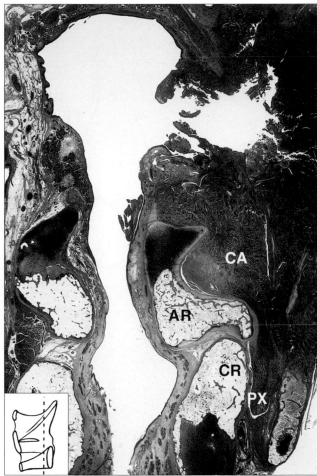

PLATE 121. Coronal section through the pyriform sinus tumor which formed the palpable mass on the anterior part of the thyroid ala. CA = cancer.

PLATE 122. Coronal section, more posterior, of the same specimen. Carcinoma (CA) impairs arytenoid (AR) movement. PX = pyriform sinus apex. CR = cricoid.

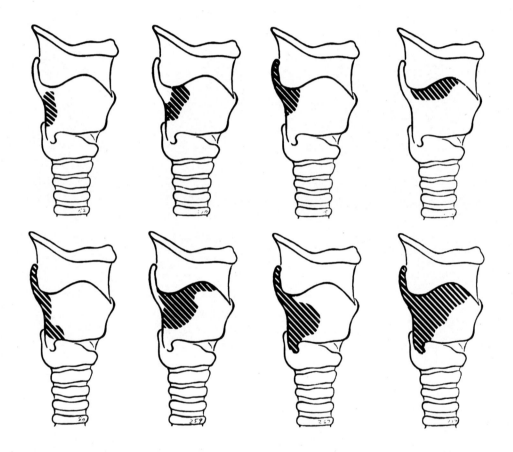

PLATE 123. Diagram showing the usual patterns of invasion into the thyroid cartilage. Survival rates for patients with cancer of the hypopharynx vary directly with invasion of the ossified laryngeal framework.[7]

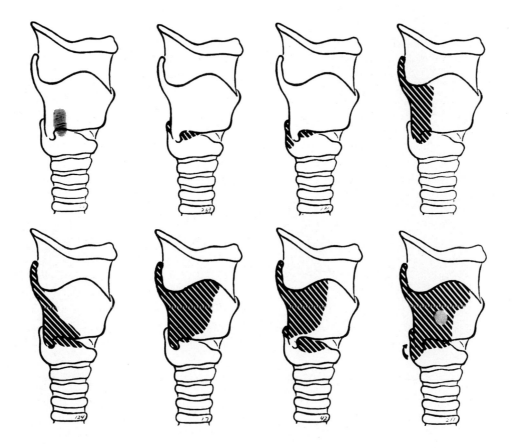

PLATE 124. Diagram showing the patterns of further invasion into the cricoid cartilage, starting at the upper ossified edge. Of 102 surgical specimens removed for pyriform sinus cancer, 38 (37%) showed invasion of the thyroid and/or cricoid cartilages.

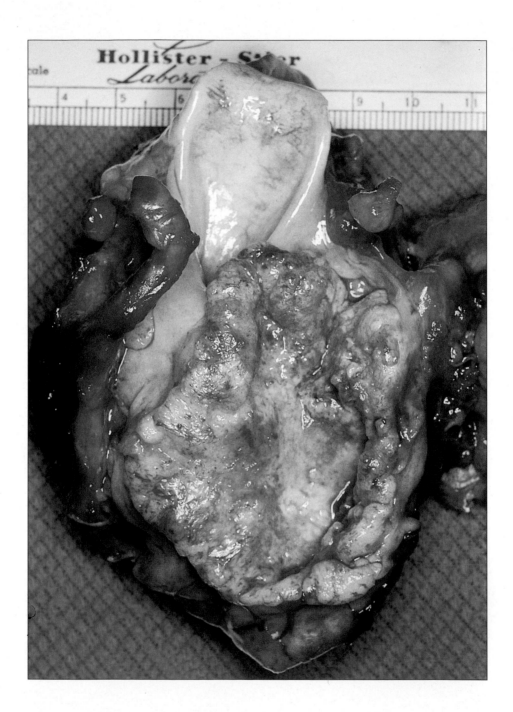

PLATE 125. Cancer of the right pyriform sinus, spreading across the cricoid plate. The right vocal cord was immobile in the paramedian position, but no intra-laryngeal tumor was seen.

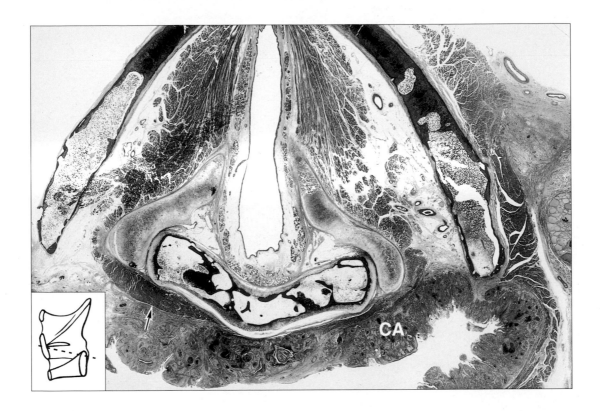

PLATE 126. Cancer has invaded the right posterior cricoarytenoid muscle at (CA). The muscle's counterpart on the left is intact, protected by its fascia (arrow).

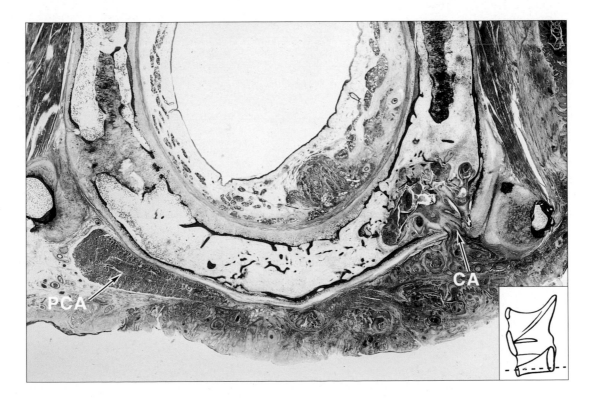

PLATE 127. Transverse section at lower level. The left PCA is still intact, while cancer (CA) has destroyed the right PCA and invaded the cricoid plate at the arrow.

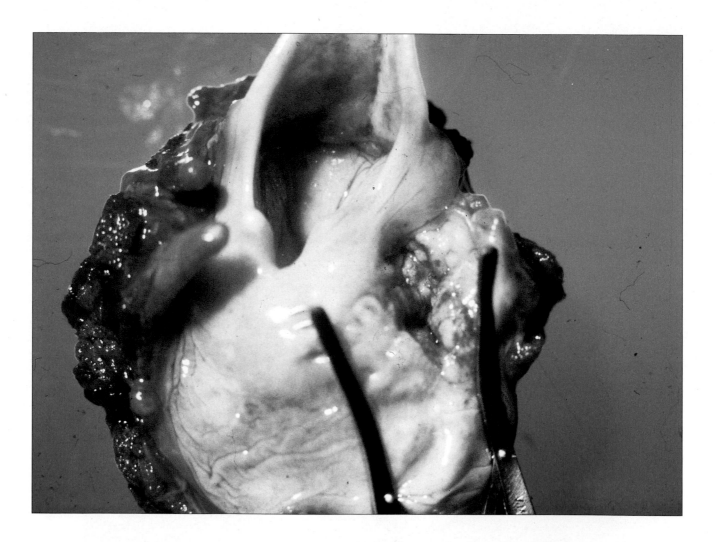

PLATE 128. Pyriform sinus cancer. The right vocal cord was immobile, but without tumor or induration.

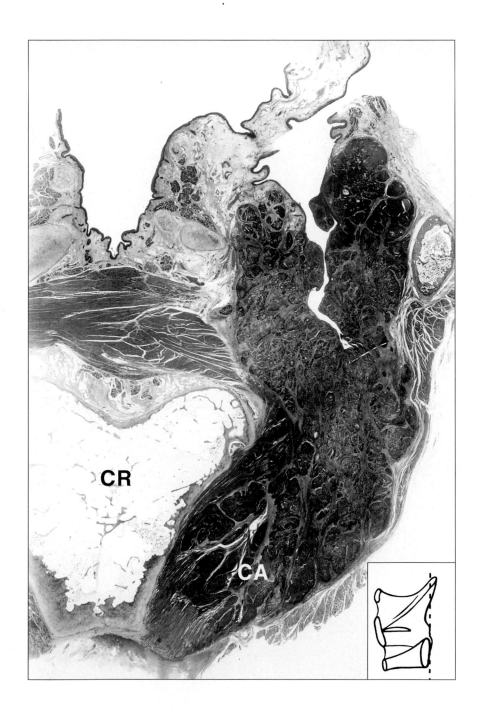

PLATE 129. Coronal section of the previous specimen. Cancer (CA) has replaced most of the right PCA muscle, destroying its power of abduction. CR = cricoid plate, posterior surface

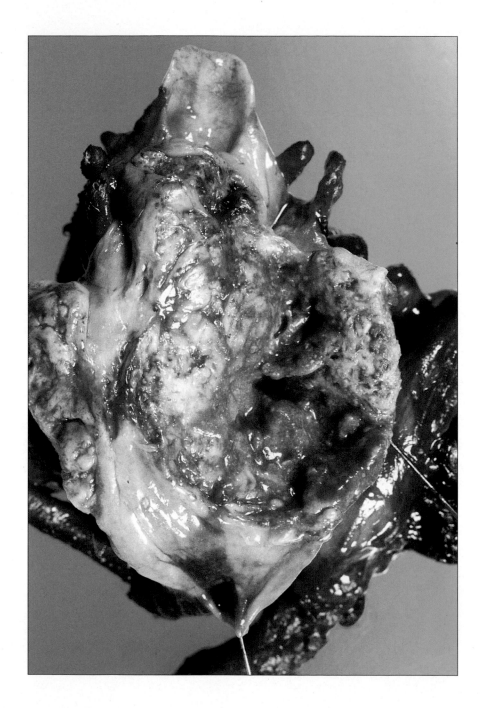

PLATE 130. Large carcinoma of the right pyriform sinus and postcricoid area. Total laryngoesophagectomy provides adequate margins and removes any "skip areas" in the esophagus below visible tumor.

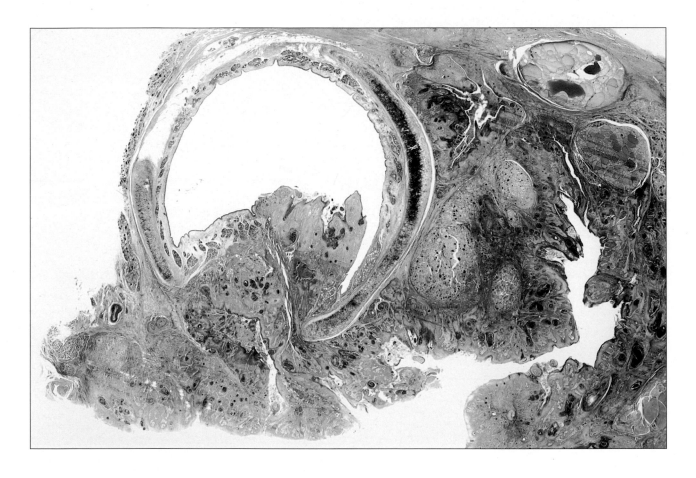

PLATE 131. Carcinoma has invaded the trachea and upper esophagus.

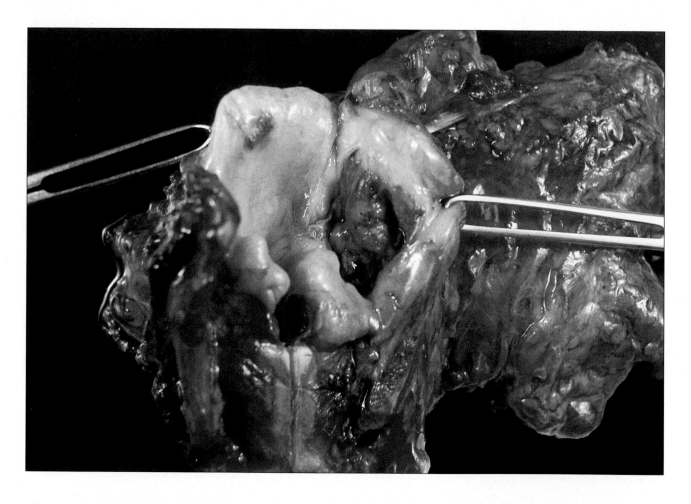

PLATES 132, 133, AND 134. Three pyriform sinus specimens treated by 4000r preoperatively during a combined treatment study. They illustrate the difficulty in assessing surgical margins at the time of operation because of edema, scar tissue, and induration.

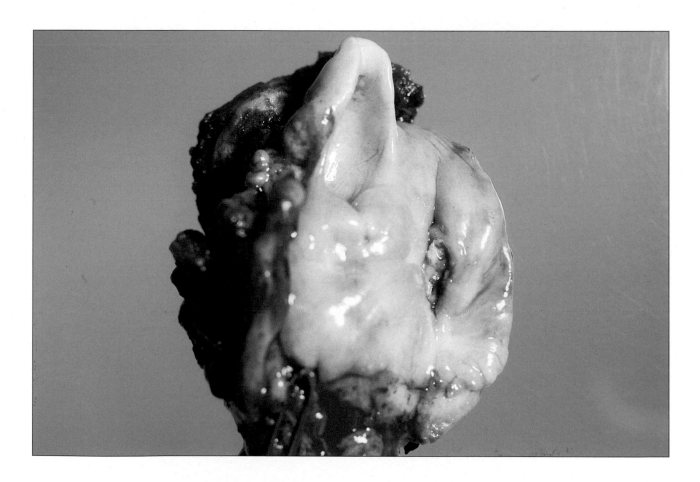

PLATE 133.

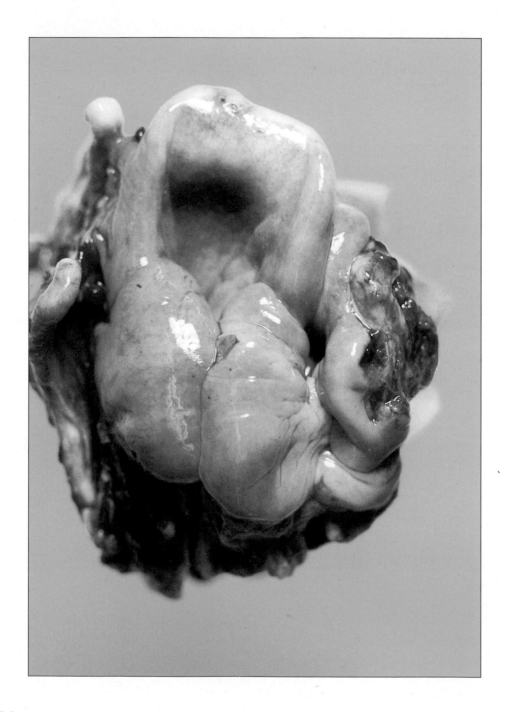

PLATE 134.

REFERENCES

1. Laccourreye O, Merite-Drancy A, Brasnu D, Chabardes E, Cauchois R, Menard M, Laccourreye H. Supracricoid hemilaryngopharyngectomy in selected pyriform sinus carcinoma staged as T2. *Laryngoscope.* 1993;103(12):1373–1379.

2. Kirchner JA. Pyriform sinus cancer: a clinical and laboratory study. *Ann Otol Rhinol Laryngol.* 1975;84:793–803.

3. Silver CE. The hypopharynx. In: Silver CE. *Surgery for Cancer of the Larynx and Related Structures.* New York: Churchill Livingstone; 1981:157–202.

4. Sato K, Kurita S, Hirano M. Location of the pre-epiglottic space and its relationship to the paraglottic space. *Ann Otol Rhinol Laryngol.* 1993;102:930–934.

5. Kirchner JA. What have whole organ sections contributed to the treatment of laryngeal cancer? *Ann Otol Rhinol Laryngol.* 1989;98:661–667.

6. Deleyiannis FW, Piccirillo JF, Kirchner JA. Relative prognostic importance of histologic invasion of the laryngeal framework by hypopharyngeal cancer. *Ann Otol Rhinol Laryngol.* 1996;105:101–108.

7. McGavran MH, Bauer WC, Ogura JH. The incidence of cervical lymph node metastases from epidermoid carcinoma of the larynx and their relationship to certain characteristics of the primary tumor. *Cancer.* 1961;14:55–66.

8. Carter D, Pipkin RD, Shephard RH, Elkins RC, Abbey H. Relationship of necrosis and tumor border to lymph node metastases and 10-year survival in carcinoma of the breast. *Am J Surg Path.* 1978;2:39–46.